Brain Surgery

A Comprehensive and Practical Resource for Brain Surgery Patients, Their Families and Physicians

Written and Illustrated by

Vini G. Khurana, M.B.B.S., B.Sc.(Med)., Ph.D.

Neurosurgeon

Bloomington, IN 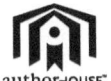 Milton Keynes, UK
authorHOUSE™

AuthorHouse™
1663 Liberty Drive, Suite 200
Bloomington, IN 47403
www.authorhouse.com
Phone: 1-800-839-8640

AuthorHouse™ UK Ltd.
500 Avebury Boulevard
Central Milton Keynes, MK9 2BE
www.authorhouse.co.uk
Phone: 08001974150

Disclaimer

While it is the intention that this book represents a comprehensive, accurate and helpful resource for persons interested in, or undergoing, brain surgery, it should be noted that the material it contains does not necessarily reflect the opinions, practices, or protocols of any given organization, institution, department, or individual. This text should be used as a useful adjunct to other available medical and educational resources related to brain disorders and their treatment. It should not be used as an alternative to personal consultation with a physician.

First published by AuthorHouse   6/17/2006

ISBN: 1-4259-2386-0 (e)
ISBN: 1-4259-2395-X (sc)

Library of Congress Control Number: 2006902181

Printed in the United States of America
Bloomington, Indiana

This book is printed on acid-free paper.

Dedication

For all the courage, sacrifices, and commitment that they share, this book is dedicated to brain surgery patients, their surgeons, and their respective families.

Acknowledgements

I thank the AuthorHouse staff for their exceptional professionalism and dedication in making this book a reality, and Mr. Chris Kontakis and his team at Ena Media for their wonderful work on **www.brain-surgery.us**, the "brain surgery help" Website.

I am deeply grateful to Doctors David Piepgras and Fredric Meyer (Mayo Clinic, Rochester, Minnesota) and Doctor Robert Spetzler (Barrow Neurological Institute, Phoenix, Arizona), the three neurosurgeons who were my extraordinary teachers.

Finally, from the bottom of my heart, I thank my parents and brother for their guidance and unreserved support, and my wife, Dianne, and daughter, Jasmine, for their precious love and spirit.

Abbreviations

3D	Three-dimensional
AD	Advance directives
ADL	Activities of daily living
AVM	Arteriovenous malformation
BBB	Blood brain barrier
BIHT	Benign intracranial hypertension
BMI	Biomedical imaging
CAT	Computer-assisted tomography
CBF	Cerebral blood flow
CBV	Cerebral blood volume
CK	Cyberknife®
CNS	Central nervous system
CPT	Chest percussion therapy
CSF	Cerebrospinal fluid
CST	Corticospinal tract
CSW	Cerebral salt wasting
CT	Computerized tomography
CTA	Computerized tomographic angiography
CTV	Computerized tomographic venography
CVA	Cerebrovascular accident
DAI	Diffuse axonal injury
DI	Diabetes insipidus
DNA	Deoxyribonucleic acid
DNI	Do not intubate
DNR	Do not resuscitate
DTI	Diffusion tensor imaging
DVT	Deep venous thrombosis
DWI	Diffusion-weighted imaging
ECG	Electrocardiogram
EEG	Electroencephalogram
ET	Endotracheal
ETV	Endoscopic third ventriculostomy
EVD	External ventricular drain
FAQs	Frequently asked questions
fMRI	Functional magnetic resonance imaging
GBM	Glioblastoma multiforme

Abbreviations (continued)

GI	Gastrointestinal
GK	Gammaknife®
GTR	Gross total resection
ICP	Intracranial pressure
ICU	Intensive care unit
IV	Intravenous
LP	Lumbar puncture
MIS	Minimally invasive surgery
MOA	Mechanism of action
MRA	Magnetic resonance angiography or arteriography
MRI	Magnetic resonance imaging
MRS	Magnetic resonance spectroscopy
MRV	Magnetic resonance venography
NF	Neurofibromatosis
NIH	National Institutes of Health
NINDS	National Institutes of Neurological Disorders and Stroke
NPH	Normal pressure hydrocephalus
OR	Operating room
OT	Occupational therapy or occupational therapist
OZ	Orbitozygomatic
PE	Pulmonary embolism
PEG	Percutaneous gastrostomy
PEJ	Percutaneous jejunostomy
PET	Positron emission tomography
PMR	Physical Medicine & Rehabilitation
POA	Power of Attorney
PT	Physical therapy or physical therapist
RN	Radiation necrosis
ROM	Range of motion
SAS	Subarachnoid space
SCD	Sequential compression device
SDH	Subdural hematoma
SIADH	Syndrome of inappropriate antidiuretic hormone secretion
SPECT	Single photon emission computed tomography

Abbreviations (continued)

SOL	Space occupying lesion
SQ	Subcutaneous
SRS	Stereotactic radiosurgery
TBI	Traumatic brain injury
TCD	Transcranial Doppler
TED	Thromboembolic disease
TIA	Transient ischemic attack
TPA	Tissue plasminogen activator
URL	Uniform resource locator
VA	Ventriculoatrial
VHL	Von Hippel Lindau
VP	Ventriculoperitoneal
VR	Virtual reality
WBRT	Whole brain radiation therapy
WHO	World Health Organization
WOS	Withdrawal of support

List of Figures

Table of Contents

CHAPTER 1.
Why does one need to know about all of this, anyway?

Brain disorders affect millions of persons worldwide. Many individuals suffering from brain tumors, brain blood vessel abnormalities, brain hemorrhage, brain trauma, hydrocephalus, and so forth, will require brain surgery to help them live. Every year in the United States of America (USA) alone, over 250,000 patients are operated on by neurosurgeons. For this reason, there arises a great need to provide more detailed, reader-friendly and practical information to the general Public regarding the many aspects of brain surgery. This book serves to address such a need.

After reading this book, the reader should have a good working knowledge of the various types of brain disorders, the way such disorders can present, the options for their investigation and treatment, and what to expect during and after treatment. Such knowledge should empower neurosurgical patients and their families with the ability to make well informed decisions along the way.

CHAPTER 2.
About the brain

Organization

The word **cerebral** refers to the brain, or **cerebrum**. The brain and spinal cord constitute the **central nervous system** (CNS). The brain is encased by a thin but tough leathery sheath or membrane known as the **dura**. Just deep to the dura is a spidery and normally watertight membrane called the **arachnoid**. Under this lies the thin **pia**, which physically coats the brain's outermost layer. The dura, arachnoid and pia are referred to as **meninges**, in that they are the three coverings or **outer barrier** of the brain (**Figure 1**).

The brain also has an important **inner barrier** known as the **blood brain barrier** (BBB). As its name suggests, the BBB exists between the blood entering the brain and the brain's nerve and supporting cell tissue. The BBB is partly formed by the cell membranes or walls of **capillary endothelial cells**, namely, the cells that line the brain's tiniest blood vessels known as **capillaries**. Endothelial cell membranes here have numerous **micropumps** and **microchannels** as well as **tight junction** bridges; all of these structures are made from proteins. The BBB is also partly formed by the **foot processes** of adjoining brain support cells known as **astrocytes**. The purpose of the BBB is to actively monitor and regulate the movement of molecules between the blood and the brain's cellular substance. BBB allows free passage of certain molecules and restricts or even blocks the movement of others as part of a key mechanism maintaining physiological equilibrium or **homeostasis**.

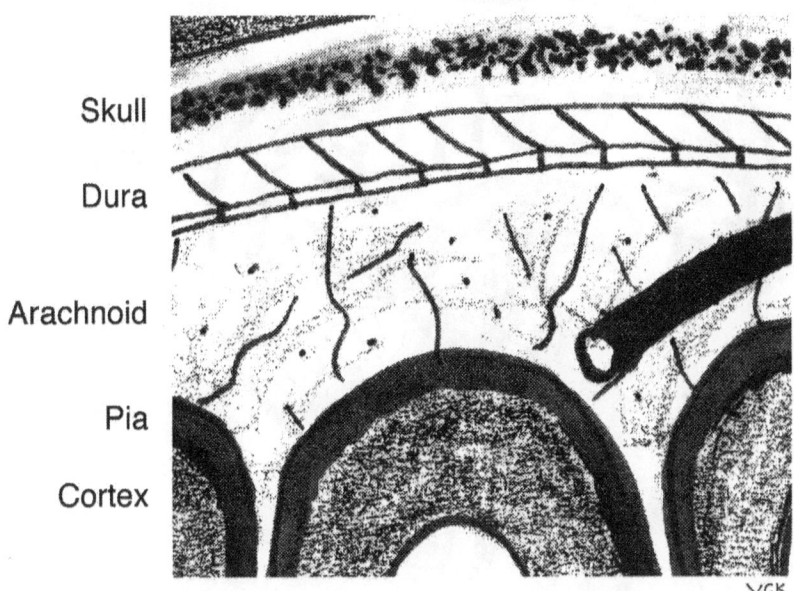

Skull

Dura

Arachnoid

Pia

Cortex

VGK

Figure 1. Coverings of the brain.

The arachnoid membrane houses the fluid surrounding the brain. This fluid, referred to as **cerebrospinal fluid** (**CSF**), lies in the **subarachnoid space** (SAS; **Figures 2 and 3**). CSF is made by small, wispy structures deep in the brain collectively called the **choroid plexus**. In adults, approximately 20 milliliters of CSF are produced each hour, and the total volume of CSF in and around the brain and spinal cord is about 125 milliliters. CSF circulates through spaces in the brain called **ventricles**, which are somewhat akin to the heart's various chambers. It exits the brain at various openings, and then circulates in the SAS both under and over the brain's outer curved surfaces or **convexities**. CSF is normally absorbed by **arachnoid granulations** which are structures that lie mainly in the midline over the convexities (**Figure 2**).

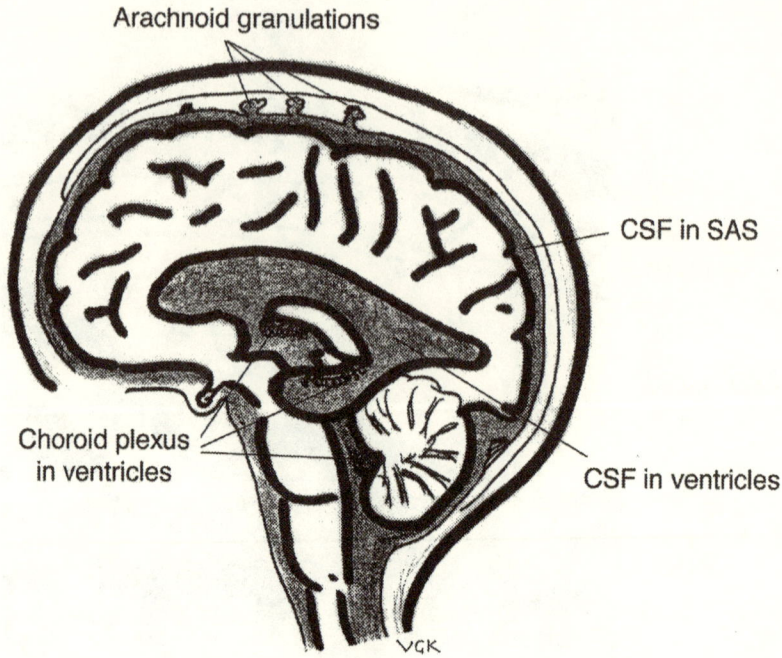

Figure 2. CSF production and absorption.

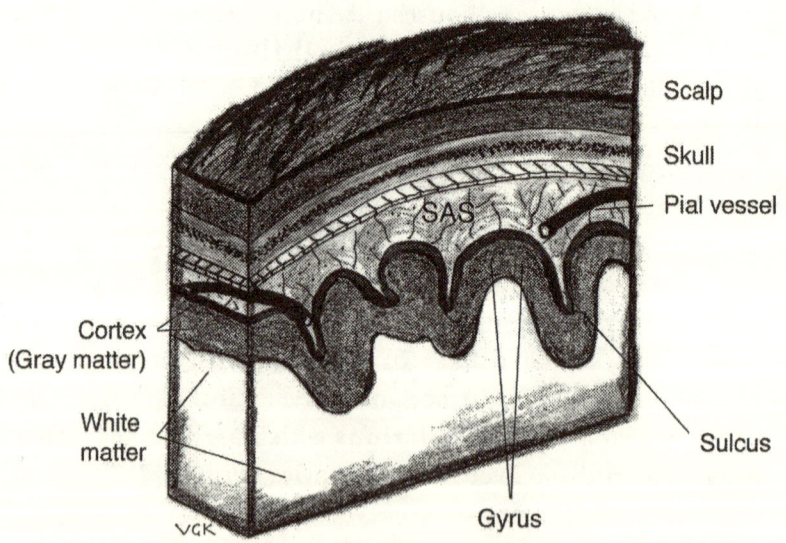

Figure 3. Brain surface.

The brain surface is referred to as the **cortex**, which means bark as in tree bark. The cortex is a few millimeters thick. The very outermost part of the cortex is referred to as the **pial surface** of the brain. In order to accommodate more of the brain's nerve cells, the cortex has many folds in it, and these are its gyri, each one being a **gyrus**. Between the gyri lie valleys or sulci, each one being a **sulcus**. In the sulci are found small blood vessels, referred to as **pial vessels (Figure 3)**.

Brain parts are often classified as **forebrain**, which is the larger upper part of the brain, and **hindbrain**, the smaller under back part of the brain (**Figure 4**). The forebrain is divided into **lobes** which include frontal, parietal, temporal and occipital (**Figure 5**), and also insular (**Figure 6**) and limbic. These are described below. The two halves of the forebrain are called **hemispheres (Figure 6)**. Interconnecting the left and right cerebral hemispheres is a dense collection of nerve fibers collectively called the **corpus callosum (Figure 7)**. The hindbrain is comprised of the cerebellum, or little brain, and the brainstem (**Figure 7**). The **cerebellum** looks like a smaller and more compact version of the forebrain, and in a brain model it appears to hang off the back undersurface of the brain, immediately behind and around portions of the brainstem (**Figure 7**). The **brainstem** is made up of, from above to below in approximate thirds, the **midbrain, pons**, and **medulla oblongata (Figure 7)**.

From the brainstem and base of the brain arise 12 pairs of **cranial nerves (Figure 7)**. These supply many structures in the head and neck. Their names (and key functions) are as follows: 1. **Olfactory** (smell); 2. **Optic** (vision); 3. **Oculomotor** (eye movement); 4. **Trochlear** (eye movement); 5. **Trigeminal** (facial sensation and chewing); 6. **Abducens** (eye movement); 7. **Facial** (taste and facial expression); 8. **Vestibulocochlear** (balance and hearing); 9. **Glossopharyngeal** (taste and throat sensation, plus gag and cardiovascular reflexes); 10. **Vagus** (voice, plus gag, cough and cardiovascular reflexes); 11. **Accessory** (neck and nape muscle function); 12. **Hypoglossal** (tongue movement).

Forebrain

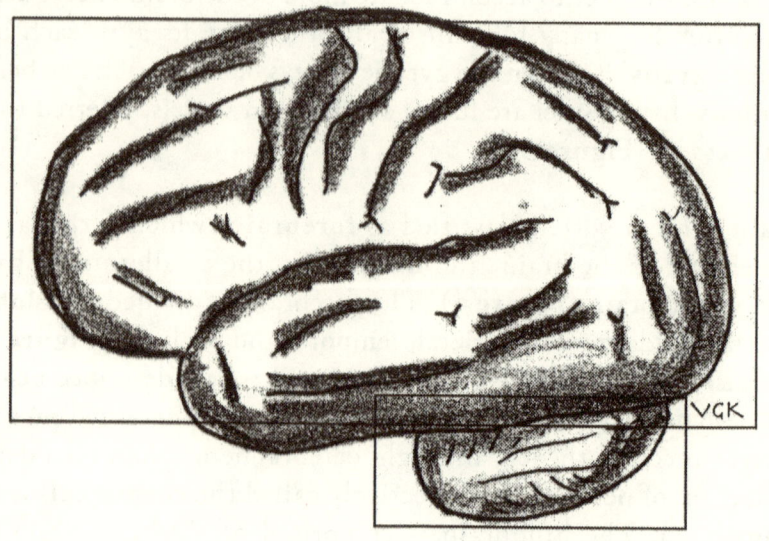

Hindbrain

Figure 4. Main subdivisions of the brain.

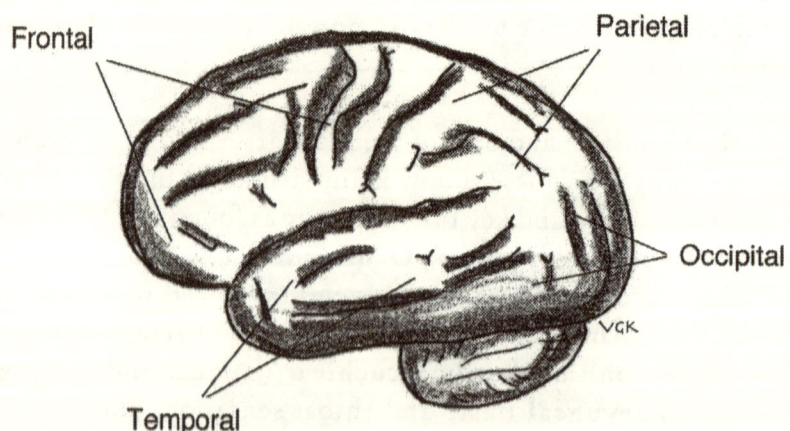

Figure 5. Lobes of the forebrain.

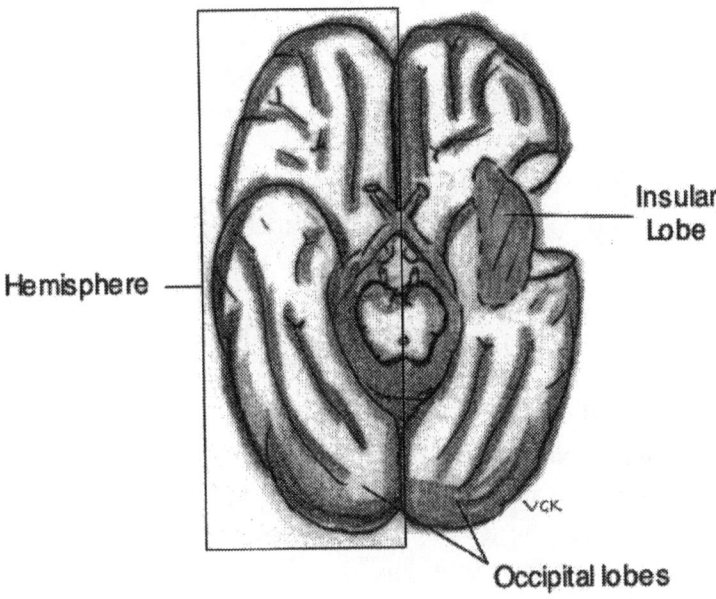

Figure 6. Forebrain hemispheres and insular lobe.

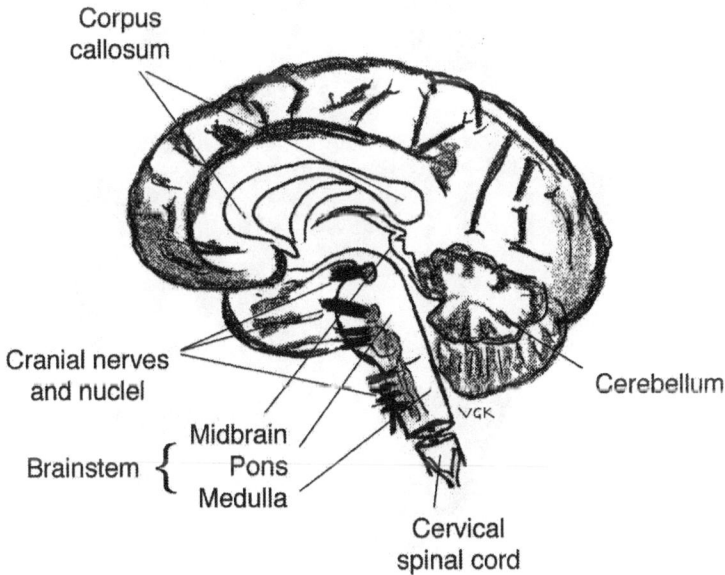

Figure 7. Corpus callosum and hindbrain.

The brain and its dura are housed in a rigid box referred to as the skull or **cranium**. There are many small openings in the base of the skull through which small blood vessels and cranial nerves pass. However, the main opening in the skull is at its base towards the back, where the bottom of the brainstem or medulla becomes the upper part of the spinal cord (**Figure 7**). This opening is called the **foramen magnum** and in adults is only three to four centimeters in diameter.

At any one time, the brain receives 20% of the heart's blood output. Regarding the organization of the brain's blood supply, there are four main pipes or trunks that enter into the brain from the neck, namely, the two **internal carotid arteries** at the front under surface of the brain and the two **vertebral arteries** at the back under surface of the brain. From the ends of these trunks arises a ring of arteries that encircles the under surface of the brain. This ring is known as the **circle of Willis (Figure 8)**. In approximately 40% of persons, this "ring" is in fact not a complete circle, a finding regarded as a normal variation of brain vessel anatomy.

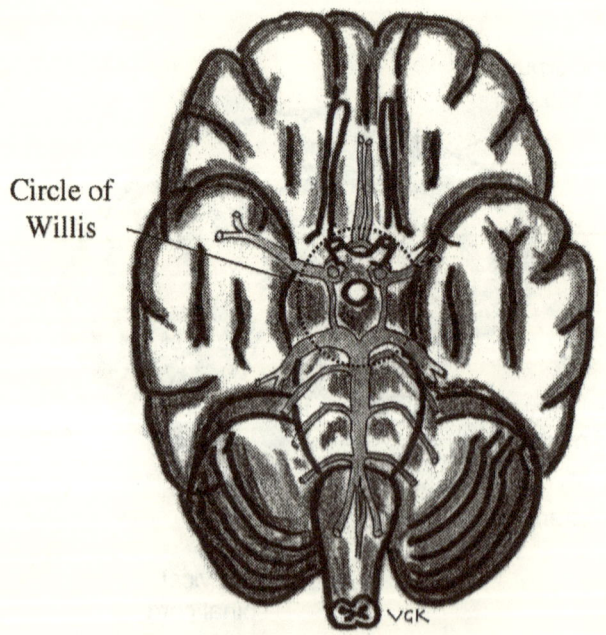

Circle of
Willis

Figure 8. Circle of Willis.

Arteries of the circle of Willis eventually give rise to **pial arteries** which course over the brain's convexities (**Figure 3**). From the pial arteries many smaller arterioles take off, usually at right angles to their parent vessels, and perforate into the brain's deeper substance. These end in capillaries, which then drain into venules and then larger veins, which then make their way into very high-volume, low-pressure venous systems known as **dural venous sinuses**. These high throughput venous channels will eventually empty into the neck's **internal jugular veins** on their way back to the heart's right atrium.

Structure

The average adult brain weighs approximately 1350 grams, or 3 pounds. It is comprised of tens of billions of cells. The vast majority of these cells are in fact not **neurons** or nerve cells, but are rather **glia** or supporting cells. Supporting cells of the brain include **astrocytes**, oligodendrocytes, microglia, ependymal cells, and others. At a microscopic level, neurons receive information at their tree-like **dendrites**, where throughput occurs at specialized structures called **synapses**. These specialized connections allow neurons to communicate by passing tiny electrical signals from one neuron to others (**Figure 9**).

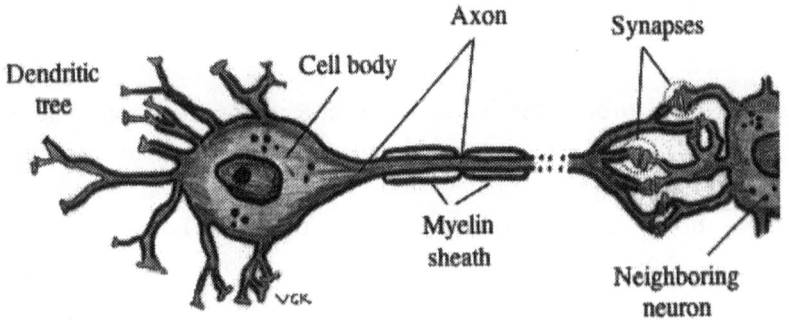

Figure 9. Neuron.

Oligodendrocytes in the brain wrap thinly layered fatty sheaths of **myelin** around **axons** which are the long electrically conductive parts of neurons. The myelin helps in maintaining the speed of electrical conduction throughout the CNS (**Figure 9**). The **gray matter** of the brain is basically its cortex and the deeper islands of neurons which form its **deep nuclei** such as the basal ganglia, thalamus, brainstem cranial nerve nuclei, and so forth. The **white matter** of the brain, which is the majority of the brain, is essentially all the myelinated pathways or **tracts** running to and from the cortex, deep nuclei, brainstem and spinal cord (**Figure 3**). The white matter also includes the corpus callosum.

Function

In essence, the left side of the brain controls the right side of the body, while the right side of the brain controls the left side of the body. For the vast majority of the population, the left hemisphere is the dominant hemisphere. **Dominance** here refers to the fact that this half of the brain is responsible for key aspects of the individual's language, memory, and higher "cognitive" functioning. While the dominant hemisphere is the left hemisphere for virtually all right-handed individuals, it may be the right hemisphere for some, but not all, left-handed individuals. The overwhelming majority of the population is right-handed and therefore left-brain-dominant.

The various lobes of the **forebrain** each subserve unique functions, but are also complexly interconnected (**Figure 10**):

- **Frontal lobe**: This is located at the upper front and midpart of the forebrain in each hemisphere, and is concerned with personality and behavior, judgment, attention, problem solving and movement planning. The primary **motor cortex** for control of the opposite side's movements from top to toe is also part of the frontal lobe. On the dominant side, which is typically the left, it also houses a critical area for speech or "expressive" language function known as **Broca's area**.
- **Parietal lobe**: This is located at the upper back and midpart of the forebrain in each hemisphere, and is concerned with the opposite side's body part sensation through the primary sensory cortex it houses. On usually the left side, it also contributes to the

ability of an individual to carry out calculations, to write, and to determine left from right. On the right side, it contributes to a person's ability to carry out certain constructional and dressing tasks, and to orient himself or herself in space.

- **Temporal lobe**: This is located at the lower midpart of the forebrain in each hemisphere, and is concerned with memory and learning, the sense of smell, and sound processing. The right temporal lobe may be more involved in visual memory, say, for faces, places, and pictures, while the left may be more involved in verbal memory, say, for names and words. On the dominant side, it houses a critical area for understanding spoken language known as **Wernicke's area.**
- **Occipital lobe**: This is located at the back of the forebrain and partly draped over the cerebellum in each hemisphere, and is responsible for processing vision. That is, actual recognition of what is seen, and associating what is seen with smells, colors, shapes, and so forth, are the critical functions of the occipital lobe.
- **Limbic lobe**: This is configured in a c-shaped manner, with the "c" cupped forward, and is located in the deeper and more inward or medial parts of each hemisphere. It is responsible for modulating a variety of emotions, including fear, rage, pleasure, feeding, laughing, and so forth. It may also play a role in motivation.
- **Insular lobe**: Like the limbic lobe, the insular lobe or insula is also hidden from view. In both hemispheres, it is an island of brain found deep to an area called the **Sylvian fissure,** where the frontal, parietal, and temporal lobes meet on the outside. The insular lobe's functions are complex and not well understood. It plays a role in taste perception, but also integrates a variety of functions spanning movement, balance, and sensation.
- **Deep nuclei**: These deep islands of nerve cells in the forebrain include the thalamus, subthalamus, caudate, putamen and globus pallidus. They collectively constitute the basal ganglia. These are responsible for the gating of movement and/or sensation for the opposite side of the body.

Regarding functions of the hindbrain (**Figure 11**):

- **The cerebellum**: This structure plays a central role in balance and coordination of movements.
- **The brainstem** and its many **cranial nerve nuclei**: These structures subserve many functions including eye movement, facial sensation and expression, chewing and swallowing, speech, hearing and balance, and contribute to head turning. Note that two cranial nerves that do not arise from the brainstem are the first and second cranial nerves, or olfactory and optic nerves, which serve the senses of smell and vision, respectively. The brainstem is also a conduit for the many long motor and sensory tracts passing to and from the brain and spinal cord. Additionally, it has major centers for the control of heart rate and breathing. That is, it houses a key **cardiorespiratory center**, in addition to centers thought to play a role in general brain activation.

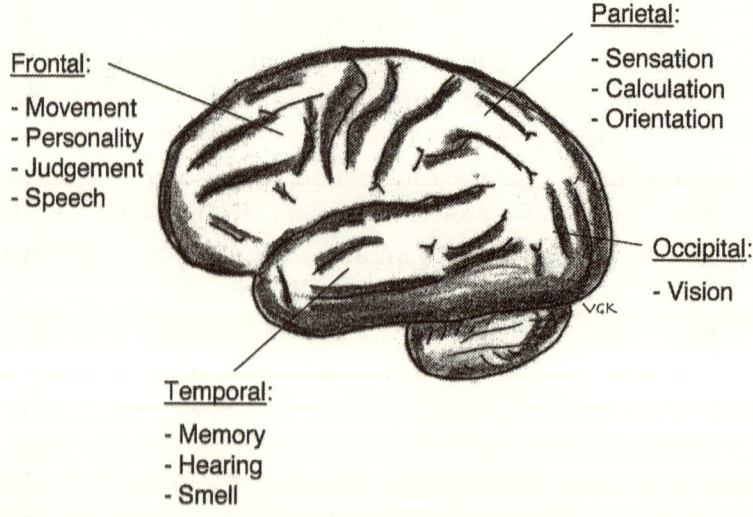

Frontal:
- Movement
- Personality
- Judgement
- Speech

Parietal:
- Sensation
- Calculation
- Orientation

Occipital:
- Vision

Temporal:
- Memory
- Hearing
- Smell

Figure 10. Forebrain functions.

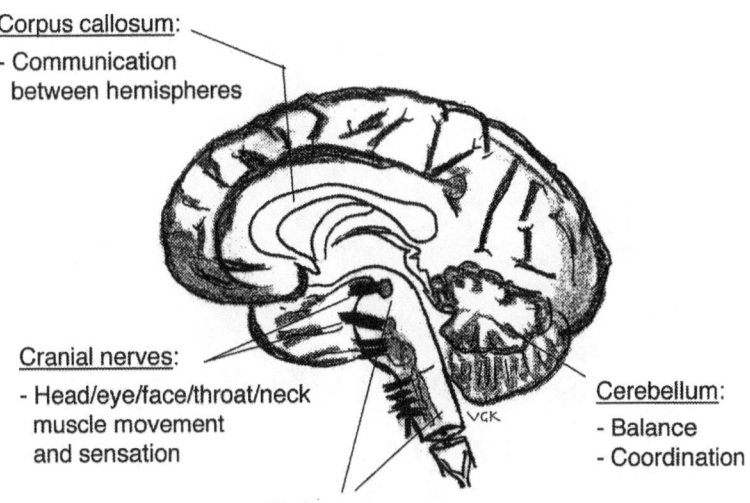

Corpus callosum:
- Communication
  between hemispheres

Cranial nerves:
- Head/eye/face/throat/neck
  muscle movement
  and sensation

Cerebellum:
- Balance
- Coordination

Brainstem:
- Cranial nerve origin
- Cardiorespiratory center
- Bridge to/from spinal cord

Figure 11. Hindbrain functions.

CHAPTER 3.
About brain surgeons

Brain surgeons, or **neurosurgeons**, are physicians who have specialized in the practice of brain surgery, or neurosurgery. After completing medical school, certain individuals apply for and are selected in neurosurgical training programs. These physicians thereby become neurosurgery "residents", or neurosurgical "trainees" or "registrars", depending on the country in which they are trained. Neurosurgery is one of the most intricate and challenging fields of medicine to learn and practice. Owing to the highly "emergent" nature of many brain disorders, the field of neurosurgery demands an extraordinary level of personal commitment to patient care.

Formal **training programs** vary in their length, but in the U.S., such programs are typically 7 years. The final year of neurosurgical residency training is referred to as the Chief Resident Year in the U.S. This is still a supervised but also more autonomous and critical year that serves as a bridge between being a neurosurgery resident-trainee and a consultant neurosurgeon. At the completion of his or her training, a neurosurgeon can elect to do one or more **Fellowships**, or none. If no fellowship is done, the neurosurgeon is a "general neurosurgeon", who may be able to surgically treat a wide variety of different disorders. However, a Fellowship is a period of time that an individual spends learning and practicing one or more particular areas of neurosurgery in greater depth. A bonafide Fellow usually travels to another institution for a year or so to acquire advanced skills under a more experienced colleague. This process is known as **subspecialization**. Neurosurgery fellowships include the following:

- **Pediatric**: Specializing in the treatment of neurosurgical disorders affecting children. This type of neurosurgeon is referred to as a pediatric neurosurgeon.
- **Cerebrovascular and skull base**: Specializing in the open surgical treatment of brain blood vessel disorders such as brain aneurysms, arteriovenous malformations (AVM), and cavernous malformations and of complex tumors occurring at the base of the skull. This type of neurosurgeon is referred to as a cerebrovascular microneurosurgeon.
- **Endovascular**: Specializing in the treatment of brain disorders through catheter-based techniques, i.e., not through open surgery. This type of neurosurgeon is referred to as an endovascular neurosurgeon. Some endovascular neurosurgeons practice both catheter-based and open surgical techniques.
- **Spine**: Specializing in the treatment of disorders of the spine and spinal cord. This type of neurosurgeon is referred to as a spinal neurosurgeon.
- **Stereotactic radiosurgery**: Specializing in the treatment of CNS disorders through focused radiation using equipment such as Gammaknife®, Linear accelerator or Linac, Cyberknife®, and so forth. This type of neurosurgeon is referred to as a stereotactic radiosurgeon.
- Other fellowships include those in **epilepsy, peripheral nerve, oncology** or CNS tumor treatment, **functional** or CNS stimulator use, and **neuroendoscopy** or microtelescope use within the CNS. There are a variety of basic sciences and clinical **research** fellowships as well, that may be incorporated into any of the above.

CHAPTER 4.
Types of brain disorders

There are a wide variety of brain disorders. Many of these require a neurosurgeon. Note that what doctors refer to as a **lesion** may be any structural abnormality such as a tumor, an inflammatory plaque, a blood clot or **hematoma**, or an aneurysm or AVM. Brain disorders can be classified as follows, with examples:

- **Vascular**: Pertaining to conditions affecting brain blood vessels. For example: Brain **aneurysms** which are balloon like outpouchings from brain vessels that can rupture or cause cerebral vasospasm following rupture (www.brain-aneurysm.com); **AVMs** which are abnormal communications between arteries and veins that can also rupture or cause seizures; **cavernous malformations** which are abnormal oozy sacs or caverns that progressively enlarge through microbleeds or microhemorrhages; and **carotid artery stenosis**, which refers to blockage of major arteries supplying the brain. Brain **hemorrhage** from uncontrolled blood pressure or **hypertension** can also occur.
- **Inflammatory**: Pertaining to conditions which cause inflammation of the brain and its coverings. For example: Neurosarcoidosis, a peculiar chronic inflammatory condition of the CNS; **vasculitis** such as giant cell arteritis or moya moya disease, referring to inflammation of blood vessel walls that can cause blood vessels to shut down or bleed as part of a stroke; and multiple sclerosis, which is a chronic disease affecting CNS nerve conduction

by damaging its white matter myelin. Also, following brain radiation, there may be some form of delayed inflammatory swelling within the brain referred to as **radiation necrosis** (RN). The swelling caused by RN can be so significant, it may be mistaken for regrowing or recurrent tumor.

- **Traumatic**: Pertaining to injury to the brain following some form of mechanical injury such as a motor vehicle accident, assault, and so forth. Some types of **traumatic brain injury** (TBI) include contusions or bruising of the brain, **subdural or epidural hematoma** which refers to an expanding collection of blood or blood clot on the brain surface, in addition to skull fractures and hemorrhage within the brain itself. A particular type of brain injury known as **diffuse axonal injury** (DAI) involves multiple areas of shear injury to brain tissue, especially axons running in the white matter, from acceleration-deceleration and torquing events.

- **Congenital**: Pertaining to conditions that an individual is born with, such as neurofibromatosis (NF), von Hippel Lindau (VHL) disease, and Chiari malformations. There may or may not be specific genetic disturbances associated with the congenital condition, and the condition itself may be diagnosed later in life when it becomes symptomatic. Certain hereditary conditions or disorders that are known to run in families due to some genetic abnormality, such as Marfan syndrome, osteogenesis imperfecta, and Ehler's-Danlos syndrome may impact upon the CNS especially through brain aneurysm formation.

- **Metabolic**: Pertaining to abnormalities of fluids and body ions or electrolytes such as **sodium**. Fluid and sodium imbalance conditions include the syndrome of inappropriate antidiuretic hormone secretion (SIADH), cerebral salt wasting (CSW), and diabetes insipidus (DI). These conditions can occur as the offshoots of other brain conditions, including TBI, brain tumors, brain surgery, and brain hemorrhage. Certain metabolic problems cause confusion or **delirium**, and can also cause **coma**. Metabolic problems causing delirium are said to be part of a metabolic encephalopathy. It should also be noted that abnormalities of **hormone** producing and releasing areas of the brain such as the hypothalamus and pituitary gland can also cause metabolic abnormalities with disturbance of body system functions. Many of these occur as a consequence of some sort of tumor or inflammatory condition affecting these critical brain areas.

- **Infective**: Pertaining to infections of the CNS. Such infections may be viral, bacterial, fungal or parasitic, depending on the bug. Such infections can cause severe inflammation of the brain and its coverings, as part of encephalitis and meningitis, respectively. Islands of pus in the brain are called **abscesses**, while a collection of pus on the surface of the brain is called an **empyema**.

- **Neoplastic**: Pertaining to tumors of the CNS. Tumors may be **primary brain tumors** such as **gliomas** or **secondary tumors** referred to as **metastases** that have spread to the CNS. Depending on their cell(s) of origin, primary CNS tumors may be classified as astrocytomas, ependymomas, Schwannomas, oligodendrogliomas, mixed oligoastrocytomas, paragangliomas, meningiomas, hemangioblastomas, germ cell tumors, lymphoma, medulloblastomas, gangliogliomas, and so forth. Such tumors may be **benign** or **malignant**, terminology that essentially reflects the speed or rate at which a tumor grows, its degree of brain-invasiveness, its curability or lack thereof, and its tendency to cause death. Examples of metastases include lung cancer and kidney or renal cancer. Interestingly, melanoma and lymphoma are examples of two tumors that can occur within the CNS as a primary tumor or can occur elsewhere in the body and spread secondarily to the CNS. Certain tumors that arise in the brain can spread or metastasize to the spinal cord or, very rarely, even spread outside of the CNS to other body organs.

- **Iatrogenic**: These are conditions that are thought to be the result of a treatment or procedure or intervention, and include wound infections, fluid overload, and other treatment-related complications.

- **Miscellaneous**: Conditions such as hydrocephalus and epilepsy are included here. **Hydrocephalus** refers to a relative increase in brain CSF, its accumulation causing a rise in brain pressure or **intracranial pressure** (ICP). A person may be born with hydrocephalus or it may occur later in life in conditions such as acquired communicating hydrocephalus, say from meningitis, and normal pressure hydrocephalus (NPH). Alternatively, obstructive or noncommunicating hydrocephalus is generally acquired in that it occurs as a consequence of some other disease process, such as a brain tumor that obstructs the normal flow of CSF in the CNS. **Epilepsy** refers to a seizure or "fit" disorder of one kind or another. Epilepsy may certainly occur as part of a congenital abnormality, or it may somehow be acquired, say in mesial temporal sclerosis, or a **seizure-generating brain tumor or AVM**.

CHAPTER 5.

Symptoms, signs and complications of brain disorders

Brain disorders can manifest in many ways. A **symptom** is a problem that a patient reports to a doctor when the doctor interviews the patient to determine his or her **medical history**. A **sign** is a problem that a doctor finds on **physical examination** of the patient. Some of the terms listed below are used to describe clusters of symptoms and signs associated with brain disorders, while others are generic or nonspecific blanket terms.

- **Neurological deficit** or **neurodeficit**: An impairment of some function of the nervous system detected by a physician.
- **Focal neurodeficit**: A specific neurological impairment that can be localized by the doctor's examination to a certain region or structure of the nervous system.
- **Paresis** and **paralysis**: Paresis refers to partial weakness on testing of a muscle group by a doctor, while paralysis or **plegia** refers to complete weakness, that is, complete loss of movement or motor activity. The following three terms are frequently used: Hemiparesis, which refers to loss of function on one side of the body; paraparesis, which refers to loss of function of the legs or lower extremities; and quadraparesis, which refers to loss of function in all four limbs, that is, both upper and lower extremities. For these three terms, if the word paresis is replaced with plegia, this refers to complete loss of movement or motor function in those parts of the body.

- **Raised ICP**: When pressure in the brain rises, say from a brain tumor, or from hydrocephalus, several symptoms can arise. There may be unexplained nausea and vomiting or headaches, particularly in the morning hours. There may be blurred or double vision, increasing drowsiness, and frank coma or unresponsiveness.
- **Brain hemorrhage**: A sudden rupture of an abnormal blood vessel, say, an aneurysm, or an AVM can cause a brain hemorrhage. The symptom is usually an **extremely severe, sudden onset headache** that may or may not be associated with a neurological deficit, neck stiffness, collapse or coma, or other signs of raised ICP.
- **"Brain Attack"** or **Stroke**: A "brain attack" is the brain's version of a heart attack, and it occurs when the blood supply to a region of the brain is lost. This is also referred to as a "stroke" or cerebral infarction or cerebrovascular accident (CVA). Symptoms of a brain attack may be short-lived, for example, less than 24 hrs in duration as occurring in a **transient ischemic attack (TIA)** or "ministroke", or they may be part of a full and permanent event, referred to as a completed stroke. Stroke symptoms are typically sudden in onset and may include one or more of the following: Visual impairment like a darkish curtain coming across the eye known as **amaurosis fugax**, or partial or complete blindness involving one or both eyes. There may be impairment of clarity of speech referred to as **dysarthria**, or language dysfunction referred to as **dysphasia** or **aphasia**. Paresis, paralysis or impaired sensation can also occur. Other symptoms include spinning or vertigo, gait imbalance, loss of consciousness, incoordination, double vision, and so forth, depending on the region of brain involved.
- **Mass effect** and **herniation**: These are important concepts that patients should be familiar with. Since the brain is enclosed in what amounts to a rigid container, the skull, there is very little room to accommodate a "**space occupying lesion**" (SOL) such as a tumor or a hematoma, or swelling in the brain referred to as **edema**. As a result, structures in the brain get compressed and begin to **shift**,

that is, they become displaced. This can lead to a wide variety of neurological symptoms and signs. This shift is known as **mass effect**. The ventricles in the brain can get compressed and trapped, and under these circumstances, CSF flow can become obstructed, leading to a further worsening of the mass effect (**Figure 12**). As the SOL or the edema associated with it continues to expand, the brain begins to be squeezed through any pathway of least resistance. This path eventually is the foramen magnum, where the critical brainstem is pushed into the spinal canal. This process of squeezing and compression is known as **herniation**, and it can progress rapidly to death (**Figure 13**). Herniating patients are often found to be progressively sleepy or "obtunded", weak or paralyzed on one side, at least one of their pupils becomes dilated and poorly reactive, and they become unable to support their breathing function.

- Miscellaneous: **Personality changes**, bladder and/or bowel incontinence, and problems with memory and thinking or **cognition** can occur in a variety of brain conditions, including tumors of the frontal lobe, dementias, and certain hydrocephalus syndromes such as NPH. Similarly, **seizures** can occur from many causes. The seizure may involve alteration in the patient's level of consciousness, where they appear blank-faced, confused or frankly unresponsive. Alternatively, seizures can involve bizarre sensory and movement or motor disturbances, or generalized shaking with potential for self injury as part of the classic "**grand mal**" or **generalized tonic-clonic seizure**.

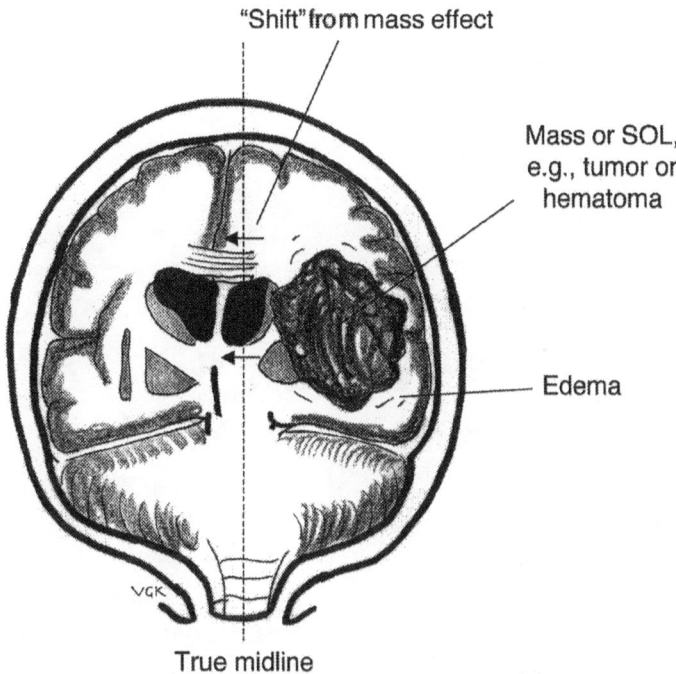

"Shift" from mass effect

Mass or SOL,
e.g., tumor or
hematoma

Edema

True midline

Figure 12. Space occupying lesion and mass effect.

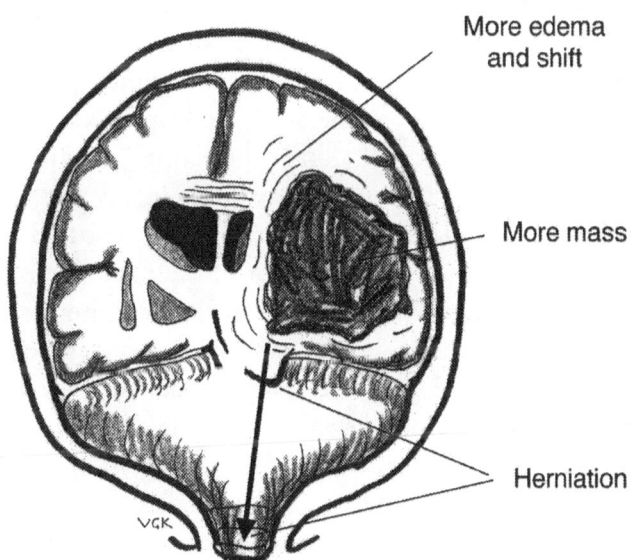

More edema
and shift

More mass

Herniation

Figure 13. Herniation.

CHAPTER 6.
Investigating brain disorders

There are many ways to investigate a brain disorder:

- **Computerized tomography** (CT) or **Computer-assisted tomography** (CAT) scanning: This technique involves a patient being put onto a sliding table and, while holding still and lying flat, being slowly advanced into a relatively wide doughnut-like scanning apparatus or **gantry**. A fast-rotating X-ray system within the gantry rapidly takes many x-rays of the patient. CT scans may be carried out with or without a **contrast agent or dye**. The use of a contrast, which is typically administered through a vein before the study, is helpful in picking up a blood vessel abnormality, or in detecting **"enhancement"** or abnormal contrast uptake and leakiness in, say, certain tumors. What CT scans lack in detail or resolution compared with other types of scans, they make up for in their speed, cost-effective convenience and **noninvasiveness**, that is, unintrusiveness. A combination of CT scanning and angiography referred to as **CT angiography** (CTA), where a larger amount of intravenous (IV) dye is introduced into the patient at the time of CT scanning, is currently gaining popularity as a very good means of detecting and characterizing blood vessel abnormalities such as aneurysms and AVMs. CTA can also be used to look at the brain's venous system, where it is referred to as **CT venography** (CTV). CTA may one day replace conventional cerebral angiography (see below), as the former is so much quicker, less expensive, and less invasive compared with the latter. Both techniques involve some degree of X-radiation, however. The ability to create high-resolution and color 3-dimensional (3D) images with CTA is very useful for surgeons planning to operate on these lesions.

- **Magnetic resonance imaging** (MRI): This technique relies on electromagnetic interaction between a large magnet and molecules within the patient's head tissues and brain. MRI scans take longer and are more expensive to obtain than CT scans, but **do not involve X-rays**, are noninvasive, and can provide very high resolution images. MRI scans, like their CT counterparts, involve the patient being slid on their backs into a doughnut-like gantry. Often, this gantry is longer and narrower than the CT's gantry, and so **claustrophobic** patients usually do not tolerate MRI scanning, although they may find it more comfortable with some form of temporary sedation. It should be noted that there are newer open MRI scanners which are uncovered on the top, and therefore less claustrophobic, however, such scanners at present don't produce very high definition studies. A well-tolerated IV contrast dye such as Gadolinium® or Magnevist® may be administered for the study. MRI scans are excellent for picking up most abnormalities of the brain, even very subtle ones. There are special forms of MRI known as **MR angiography** or arteriography (MRA) and **MR venography** (MRV) that are designed to look specifically at brain arteries and veins, respectively. These are being developed to perhaps replace formal catheter cerebral angiography (see below) as MRA and MRV, like CTA and CTV, are noninvasive ways at looking at brain blood vessels. MRA and MRV techniques are used in **screening** for brain aneurysms and AVMs. A special MR sequence known as **diffusion-weighted imaging** (DWI) is used to detect strokes, certain tumors and infections, DAI, and so forth. Finally, another special form of MRI known as **MR spectroscopy** (MRS) is being developed as a noninvasive technique to detect the spectroscopic pattern or biochemical signatures of certain molecules in the brain, and lesions within the brain. It may be helpful in determining the more exact location of a tumor cell mass or differentiating regrowth or recurrence of certain tumors from post-radiation change or infection.

- **Cerebral angiography:** Cerebral angiography involves injection of an opaque dye into the blood stream of a patient. The injection is made through a **catheter** or thin piece of tubing inserted into, and advanced towards the neck from, the femoral artery in the groin area (**Figure 14**). The dye eventually reaches the brain circulation, and X-rays are taken at this point. The dye is "radio-opaque" in that X-rays don't pass as easily through it as they do through neighboring brain tissue, so the dye stands out. This way, a roadmap of the brain circulation is obtained, telling a physician about the state of the arteries and veins in terms of their course, their pattern of communication, their diameters and lengths, and any other abnormalities. The abnormal blush or sometimes rich blood supply of a tumor may be seen, or an aneurysm or AVM detected and characterized. At present, cerebral angiography remains the best method or "**gold standard**" investigation for brain aneurysms and AVMs. Arteries in spasm, say following rupture of a brain aneurysm, can be detected and potentially treated using catheter angiography techniques.

- **Positron emission tomography** (PET) scanning: This technique involves IV injection or inhalation of a small and safe dose of **radioactive tracer**. As the tracer decays, its presence and location are detected by a special PET camera. Although PET scanning does not provide a highly detailed or high-resolution map of the body part scanned, it does provide potentially useful information. Further, PET images can be overlapped or **coregistered** with brain MRI or CT images from the same patient to provide a more detailed "functional" map of the patient's brain. PET imaging data collected by the computer can allow a physician to tell, say, whether there is impaired **blood flow** to the regions of a patient's brain, or if there is **metastatic tumor** present in different parts of the patients body, or whether the abnormality detected on the MRI of a brain tumor patient who has received radiation therapy is **regrowth of tumor versus radiation-related change**. Some limitations of PET are that it is a costly technique which relies on highly advanced technology and considerable expertise to interpret the data accurately. As a result, not all medical facilities have a PET scanner.

- **Single photon emission computed tomography** (SPECT) scanning: SPECT scanning is somewhat like PET scanning in the way it works, except that it provides information more exclusively on **cerebral blood flow** (CBF) and cerebral blood volume (CBV). Again, a small and safe amount of IV or inhaled **radioactive tracer** is administered to the patient to acquire this data. The technique is excellent for looking at **CBF impairment**, and for assessing for location of **seizure activity** "hot spots" in epilepsy patients. Just as for PET, the SPECT images can be "fused" with brain MR images from the same patient, that is, MR-SPECT. SPECT imaging shares the same limitations as PET, and as a result is not available at all medical facilities.

- **Ultrasound techniques**: Ultrasound techniques such as duplex or Doppler presently play no major role in the detection of brain conditions except in the setting of TIA or stroke from carotid or neck artery blockage or stenosis. Here, the ultrasound probe placed along the neck skin can be used to detect the degree of blockage and alteration in blood flow velocity across the narrowed segment. Sometimes, a small ultrasound probe is used during open brain surgery to confirm that there is good blood flow in an artery, say, after a brain aneurysm coming off the side of that vessel has been clipped or after brain bypass (www.brain-aneurysm.com). In patients who have experienced rupture of a brain aneurysm, a potentially serious complication known as cerebral vasospasm can develop (www.brain-aneurysm.com). Here, an ultrasound technique called **transcranial Doppler** (TCD) can be used to screen patients at the bedside for the development of vasospasm. In TCD, a small ultrasound probe is gently pressed against regions of the scalp, and a signal related to brain artery blood flow is picked up and analyzed.

- **Lumbar puncture** (LP): The goal of carrying out an LP is to obtain fluid from a CSF-filled pouch called the **lumbar cistern** located deep to the soft tissue and spinolaminar bone of the lower back in the midline. A spinal needle is used for this, and it is inserted using local anesthetic to numb the skin and underlying tissues. There may be some tugging, but it should not be painful. Usually about 5-10 milliliters of CSF are removed. An LP can yield a lot of useful information regarding brain conditions. For example, CNS **infection**, MS, and certain tumors such as germ cell tumors and lymphomas frequently leave "footprints" that can be detected in the CSF. The **pressure** at which the CSF is under can be detected via an LP, and this information can be used to help diagnose conditions such as benign intracranial hypertension (BIHT) or pseudotumor cerebri, and other conditions involving hydrocephalus. Sometimes, a significant volume of CSF can be removed as part of a "large-volume spinal tap" to help physicians determine if a patient with BIHT or with NPH improves in his or her symptoms. Additionally, subtle amounts of blood that may not be seen on a CT scan following, say, rupture or leak of a brain aneurysm, may in fact be detected using an LP. Here, examination of the CSF for blood pigments or "**xanthochromia**" is carried out.

- **Blood tests**: Taking a small sample of blood from a vein may be useful in the setting of following a patient for infection or inflammation that may be affecting a surgical wound, blood stream, brain tissue, brain blood vessels, and so forth. For patients with **fluid and electrolyte imbalance**, blood sodium and blood concentration or osmolality can also be assessed this way. Some genetic mutations and variations known as **polymorphisms** that are associated with certain CNS disorders can be picked up by screening the deoxyribonucleic acid (DNA) present in the patient's white blood cells (www.brain-aneurysm.com).

• **Brain biopsy**: At times, a sample of brain and meningeal tissue may be needed to help diagnose a condition whose diagnosis cannot otherwise be reliably made by the tests described above. An operation is required. The operation may involve open surgery or insertion of a needle-like brain probe to take a sample of brain tissue. The former is referred to as craniotomy for open biopsy, while the latter is referred to as stereotactic brain needle or core biopsy (**Chapters 12 and 13**).

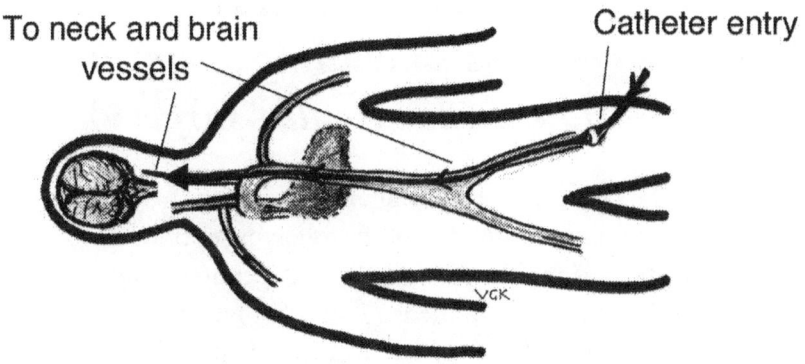

To neck and brain vessels

Catheter entry

Figure 14. Cerebral angiography.

CHAPTER 7.

Treatment options (including open surgery, radiation, endovascular surgery)

There are several treatment or "**management**" options for patients with conditions affecting the brain. Any of the following options may be used alone or in combination. The option(s) used depend(s) largely upon the type of condition, but may also depend on other factors such as the age and medical condition of the patient. Management options include:

- **Observation**: When a patient's lesion is observed, this implies that **no active treatment** is undertaken. However, over time, a physician typically follows the patient by periodic brain imaging and by history and physical examination to determine whether the lesion is becoming worthy of treatment. Such a determination may be made by the fact that the lesion is growing, or now causing symptoms. Each of the following examples may involve situations where no treatment is advised or requested. However, it should be noted that the decision to treat or not to treat is one usually made in joint consultation with the patient, and his or her family and physicians, and it is made on a case-by-case basis. Examples include: (1) A benign brain tumor called a meningioma can be followed by periodic scans if this lesion is small and not causing any symptoms; (2) a small, smooth looking brain aneurysm in a patient with no family history of brain aneurysms and no personal history of other brain aneurysms, can also be followed with periodic scans if deemed suitable by the physician; (3) an elderly patient with multiple medical problems and a newly diagnosed malignant brain tumor may elect to not undergo any treatment for the condition, or the patient and family may request this; (4) the family of a patient who is comatose from a massive brain hemorrhage may elect not to pursue any active treatment of the patient in line with the patient's wishes and the likelihood of no benefit from intervention for that particular patient. In such cases, the decision to observe as opposed to treat may be made because the treatment option for that particular patient is thought to be of excessive risk relative to benefit, or of no anticipated benefit.

- **Medical management**: The medical treatment of a patient involves administration of medications such as steroids, anti-seizure medications, pain medicines, blood thinning agents, anti-inflammatory medications, and/or the use of physical therapy. Note that **steroids** are a class of medications administered orally or IV with the aim of reducing a particular type of brain swelling referred to as **vasogenic edema**. Steroid therapy is commonly used in patients with primary and metastatic brain tumors, and may be for several days to several weeks. Steroids may also be given to tumor patients prior to or during brain radiation. Finally, regarding medically managed patients, the physician may have counseled a patient that the medical option is to be tried before the surgical option, or that the surgical option is not appropriate for the treatment of that condition in that particular patient. Again, this decision is made on a case-by-case basis.

- **Open surgery**: Open surgery or operative neurosurgery involves some form of operation or neurosurgical procedure. This may be a **craniotomy**, or a brain biopsy, placement of an external ventricular drain (EVD) or shunt, and so forth. These are discussed in detail elsewhere (**Chapters 12 and 13**). If the decision is to undergo open surgery, the benefits of this treatment option should outweigh its risks. Conditions requiring open surgery can include brain aneurysms, brain tumors, expanding brain blood clots or hematomas, hydrocephalus, and so on.

- **Radiation and radiosurgery: Whole brain radiation therapy** (WBRT), as the name implies, involves administration of some form of radiation to the patient's brain. It is generally a painless procedure that is typically undertaken in **fractions** or portions over several weeks under the supervision of a radiation oncologist. **Radiosurgery** also involves some form of radiation, except that it is usually administered on a single day in one dose, and is very focused in that it targets a very specific part of the patient's brain, usually a region somewhere between 1-3 cm in diameter. Owing to its focused nature, it is called **stereotactic radiosurgery** (SRS). This is discussed in detail elsewhere (**Chapter 14**). Radiation is administered mainly for tumors, and usually after surgery has been carried out. However, some blood vessel abnormalities and painful conditions such as trigeminal neuralgia may be amenable to radiosurgery, among other treatment options.

- **Endovascular surgery:** Endovascular surgery involves an endovascular surgeon or interventional neuroradiologist using a catheter, as described for cerebral angiography (**Chapter 6**), to navigate to a part of the patient's blood vessel tree and carry out treatment of a brain abnormality such as a brain aneurysm, AVM, or very vascular brain tumor. Endovascular surgery is described elsewhere (**Chapter 15**). During endovascular surgery, the catheter can be used to deliver or deploy a variety of devices and compounds such as: (1) A **contrast dye** which lights up the patient's vascular tree; (2) one or more soft, flexible **platinum microcoils** that fill the sac of a brain aneurysm to slow the blood flow within this lesion and cause it to clot off; (3) a **balloon** to widen a blood vessel that is in spasm, a procedure called **angioplasty**; (4) a **stent** left in the blood vessel. A stent is basically an expansile hollow bridge that can keep a narrowed blood vessel open, or through which microcoils may be deployed into, say, the sac of a brain aneurysm. Additionally: (5) A "vasodilating" medication such as **papaverine** or a calcium channel blocking agent such as **verapamil**, which can cause a blood vessel in spasm to open up again; (6) a **glue** or resin or an equivalent "polymerizing compound" that can be squirted through the catheter directly into, say, a highly vascular tumor or complex AVM to shut down its blood supply; (7) a blood clot dissolving or "**thrombolytic**" medication such as **tissue plasminogen activator** (TPA) which can be used in some patients within a few hours of sudden stroke to dissolve the blood clot and perhaps restore blood flow to the patient's brain. Again, the decision to undergo endovascular surgery implies that the benefits of this treatment option outweigh its risks, and endovascular surgical procedures may be carried out alone or, for example, before or after an open surgical procedure.

- **Chemotherapy**: Chemotherapy medications tend to target rapidly dividing cells found in high-grade tumors or cancers. There are many different compounds that are each referred to as chemotherapy agents, many combinations, and many different **mechanisms of action** (MOA). These medications are usually administered IV or orally, usually for months and commonly in several separate stretches or "cycles". Sometimes they are delivered directly into the CSF, say, through an Ommaya reservoir (**Chapter 13**), or they may be implanted into the brain tumor itself as a group of small "wafers". It is beyond the scope of this book to describe the many agents, their MOA and recommendations for their administration. Resources detailing these are given elsewhere (**Chapter 24**).

Potential complications of the main treatment options are described elsewhere (**Chapters 16 and 18**).

CHAPTER 8.
What a patient should think about

There are many things to consider for a patient diagnosed with a brain condition.

Has the patient been presented with a complete and balanced picture about treatment options?

The various treatment options have been detailed in the preceding chapter.

Will the patient have the option of being treated at an experienced center by an experienced group of doctors?

Safe and effective brain surgery requires a neurosurgeon with the appropriate training for that condition, and a sophisticated and dedicated **neurological intensive care unit** (ICU) and neuro-ICU service. It is indisputable that brain conditions typically require expert attention and a strong commitment by physicians and patients alike to both initial care and follow-up. It is now becoming apparent in the literature that the successful treatment of certain brain conditions is helped significantly by the availability of **hospital resources** including appropriate intraoperative equipment, endovascular and radiosurgical suites, neuro-ICU, and suitably trained nursing and paramedical personnel. All of this in addition to a team of appropriately trained and experienced **specialists** including microneurosurgeons, endovascular surgeons, radiosurgeons, and neurocritical care "intensivists". Such resources and staff should be found at most large **teaching or "tertiary referral" centers**, but may also be found in certain regional "private" practices and their associated hospitals. Wherever and whenever possible, it behooves a patient to **check with the physician** regarding the neurosurgeon's experience with that particular condition, the number of patients with that condition he or she treats every year, and the sophistication of the hospital facility, including the mandatory presence of a neuro-ICU.

What is the best treatment for a particular lesion?

The following discussion does not focus on a specific brain condition, but rather conveys general points that apply to the diverse family of brain lesions.

- **Lesion-specific factors**: These include the size of the lesion, the rate at which it is growing which may or may not be known, its specific location in the brain and its relationship to neighboring critical blood vessels, cranial nerves, and so forth. The anticipated type of lesion, based on its imaging features, may also be a factor when considering treatment options.
- **Physician-specific factors**: The superspecialized training of the neurosurgeon, the surgeon's judgment, and his or her experience are intuitively important in determining the outcome of brain surgery. It is frequently difficult for a patient to figure these things out in advance. The Internet may be of some assistance, but frequently it boils down to local hearsay, direct questioning, and trust.
- **Technology-specific factors**: The art and science of open brain surgery is a time-tested and potentially effective treatment. There are decades of data regarding its safety and efficacy in the setting of a variety of brain conditions. Open surgery is of course not without risk. No open or endovascular surgical or radiosurgical intervention carries zero risk. Endovascular surgery and SRS are often "sold" as "no incision, no open operation, and a short or no hospital stay", and this is for the most part true unless a complication arises and a microneurosurgeon's assistance is

required. While many microneurosurgeons have been able to minimize "head shaves", they have not been able to eliminate the need for an incision, open operation, and hospitalization. Further, the long-term effectiveness of endovascular surgery and SRS for many neurosurgical conditions remains to be established.

- **Patient-specific factors**: A patient may choose to have one form of treatment over another regardless of counseling. For example, a patient may flatly refuse any type of open surgery and opt for endovascular or radiosurgical treatment, which may indeed work out just fine for certain conditions. On the other hand, some patients simply "want it taken care of" by open surgery, that is, without the burden of additional uncertainty and prolonged followup which can occur with SRS and endovascular surgery in certain situations. A patient's advanced age and poor medical condition may make attempted endovascular or radiosurgical treatment a safer option, in the hope that an operation, general anesthetic and longer postoperative ICU stay can be avoided for such patients.

- **Medical facility-specific factors**: A brain surgery patient's outcome may, in part at least, be related to the hospital at which the patient presents based merely on geographic proximity. As elaborated earlier, the availability of a 24-hour on-call highly specialized medical team is the hallmark of what is required to give such patients their best chance of a good outcome. Fortunately, such teams are usually present in large teaching hospitals. These centers will typically be able to offer endovascular, radiosurgical, and open surgical treatment options, and should be able to have discussed among several colleagues in a **multidisciplinary** manner those more complex neurosurgery cases for which a consensus opinion regarding best possible treatment is sought.

- **Media-specific factors**: Media hype is a factor influencing treatment considerations. Members of the media may look at a new technology as a breakthrough without a deeper understanding of how the technology may translate to patient care, and how individualized and comprehensive an analysis of a neurosurgery patient should be. Unless opinions related to the technology are sought from a multitude of experienced physicians, including those of different neurosurgical subdisciplines, the potential to introduce bias into such reports remains high.

- **Medical industry-specific factors**: Developing new technologies that may impact upon hundreds of thousands of persons worldwide every year is potentially lucrative. Large companies may have invested a lot of time and money on technology research and development, and they understandably want it to pay off. That is not to say that the technology may not work or be suitable. It may indeed be excellent for many neurosurgery patients with that condition. However, it is unlikely to be suitable for all patients with that condition. One should be aware of "**conflicts of interest**" and any hidden agenda of "big business" or "self-interest" groups.

CHAPTER 9.

What a surgeon may be thinking about

As **William J. Mayo**, one of the founders of the Mayo Clinic stated: *"The best interest of the patient is the only interest to be considered."* When it comes to a patient with a brain lesion, the following must be carefully considered:

- **For symptomatic lesions**: The lesion may be causing neurological problems or complaints in the patient such as headaches, seizures, cranial nerve palsies or dysfunction, limb weakness, imbalance, impaired or double vision and other sensory disturbances, and hydrocephalus. After a careful history, physical examination and appropriate studies (**Chapter 6**) are obtained, the physician should be able to determine if the lesion is symptomatic or not. If it is symptomatic, treatment is favored.
- **For asymptomatic lesions**: A physician may elect to observe an asymptomatic lesion, and will generally arrange for periodic brain imaging and Office visits to assess if the lesion is becoming symptomatic. However, even if it is not causing any neurological disturbance, treatment of an asymptomatic lesion may still be recommended if the lesion is enlarging or of a worrisome type, size, shape or location.
- **The patient's history**: For example, if the patient has a personal history of rupture from a previous separate brain aneurysm, or a family history of aneurysmal rupture, or an inherited connective tissue disorder that predisposes towards the growth

of brain aneurysms, treatment of a newly diagnosed aneurysm in that patient may be favored, even if it is a smaller one (www. brain-aneurysm.com).

- **The treatment option(s)**: The rationale for which treatment(s) to offer varies according to many factors (**Chapters 7 and 8**). These factors should be carefully weighed by the treating physician(s), and decisions made on an individualized or "**case-by-case**" basis. This involves appropriate discussion with the patient, and possibly also with medical colleagues of the treating physician, particularly if the condition is a complex one.

CHAPTER 10.
Informed consent

Informed consent is the process by which the physician communicates relevant and accurate information to the patient and his or her family members prior to carrying out a procedure. It is not a one-way communication, but rather a time where the questions and concerns of the patient and family members can also be addressed.

The neurosurgeon should be expected to obtain informed consent from the patient before proceeding with any form of treatment. During a brain surgery patient's investigation and treatment process, other procedures that a patient may encounter requiring informed consent include, but are not limited to, cerebral angiography, LP, and placement of an EVD, lumbar drain or CSF shunt. Additionally, the patient or his or her family members may be asked to enroll in a relevant clinical trial or study. This, too, requires informed consent to be obtained.

Informed consent should of course include an honest and candid discussion of the **risks and expected benefits** of the procedure, and a **description** of the planned procedure. At the end of this discussion, one should be able to clearly weigh in one's mind whether the procedure's benefits outweigh its risks, which is the usual expectation. Another topic that should be discussed in a comprehensive informed consent is any **appropriate alternative(s)** to the proposed procedure. For example, observation of the lesion versus surgery or, where appropriate, biopsy of a lesion versus an attempt at its complete removal or resection, and so forth. Informed consent should also include mention of a **team approach**. Assisting the attending surgeon may be a neurosurgeon-in-training, that is, a neurosurgical "Resident", "Chief Resident" or "Registrar", or a "Fellow". Finally, informed consent for neurosurgery should include a question by the doctor regarding the patient's "**advance directives**" (AD). That is, does the patient have a Living Will or other written directive that informs the health care team and family members alike regarding the patient's wishes should he or she at some point become unable to communicate those wishes? The physician should document all of the above, in addition to the procedure he or she has been given permission to carry out, including **which side of the head**. A final statement regarding the fact that the patient and his or her family members agree to the above and wish to proceed with the discussed procedure should also be documented.

In summary, a **comprehensive informed consent** includes a discussion of the following elements:

- Benefits of the procedure
- Risks of the procedure
- Overview of the planned procedure
- Alternatives to the procedure
- Team approach
- Advance directives
- The anticipated type, side and date of the procedure
- The desire to proceed as discussed

Note that there are certain situations where a patient cannot provide informed consent. For example, a **minor**, not of legal adult age, which is typically 18 years. Here the parents should be able to provide informed consent. Alternatively, a patient may have some form of significant **cognitive or mental impairment**, that is, he or she may be confused, comatose, demented, or significantly mentally challenged. The hospital facility should have guidelines regarding how to obtain consent in these special circumstances, and regarding how to provide care deemed medically necessary and in the best interests of the patient. In a life-threatening emergency such as a hospital receiving a comatose ruptured aneurysm or herniating patient upon whom medical personnel need to carry out a potentially life-saving procedure but are unable to contact the patient's family members and have no AD, the best interests of the patient should be the only consideration. In such a circumstance, two or more physicians may fulfill the requirements for **emergency consent**, and generally proceed to do what they were trained to do: heal the sick and save lives.

CHAPTER 11.
Preparing for open surgery

The **perioperative** period is a time involving the few days before and after open surgery. The **preoperative** period is before surgery, while the **postoperative** period is after. In the preoperative period, a patient should have met the microneurosurgeon who will carry out the surgery. The discussions should have involved some of the topics covered in the preceding chapters. The patient may also have met a member of the **anesthesia team** involved in administering a general anesthetic to the patient and looking after the patient during the operation itself. The surgeon should have discussed the benefits, risks, alternatives and team approach for surgery (**Chapter 12**), reviewed the basics of the surgery and recovery period, and addressed any questions or concerns that the patient may have. The anesthesiologist will want to know the patient's basic medical history, medications, allergies, any previous anesthetics, and so forth. For **elective brain surgery**, that is, surgery planned in advance by the surgeon and patient to be carried out on a certain date, a patient may have to undergo routine blood tests, chest x-ray and electrocardiogram (ECG) testing to be formally cleared for surgery. Any further testing and consultation depends on the medical condition of the patient, but for most patients, the process of preoperative workup is fairly straightforward and brief. A patient should tell his or her doctor if taking **medications that can thin the blood** such as Coumadin/Warfarin, Plavix, Ticlid, and Aspirin.

The evening before surgery, a patient should have a good meal and get some rest. Usually from midnight onwards on that night before surgery, the patient should not eat or drink anything, however one should check with the doctor regarding taking any regular medications. On the morning of surgery, or at the time prearranged by the doctor's Office staff with the patient, the patient should make his or her way to the admitting area of the hospital. The admitting staff will assist patients and their families. They will generally confirm a patient's identity, the side on which the operation is to be carried out, that is, left versus right, and answer any questions or concerns before surgery. They may confirm if the patient has an AD with them, such as a Living Will or another equivalent document.

CHAPTER 12.

The open surgical procedure and early postoperative period

Most brain surgeries take about 3-5 hours of operating time. However, by the time a patient has been called down to surgery, administered general anesthesia, operated on, woken up following surgery, observed in the postoperative recovery area, and then transferred to the ICU, many more hours may pass. It is normal for family members to be anxious during times of surgery on a loved one, and there is generally a waiting area in the ICU or near the operating room (OR) complex to which family members will be directed. If family members leave that area, they should leave a contact number with the staff there so that they can be reached, even if only for an update regarding how the surgery is proceeding. Not all institutions have "**Communicators**" who provide periodic updates during the surgery. Also, it is important to note that some brain surgeries may take longer owing to the complexity of the lesion or if there is more than one lesion being treated. This is generally discussed by the neurosurgeon prior to elective surgery. A neurosurgeon will take "**as long as it takes**" to carry out the surgery as skillfully and as safely as possible. The neurosurgeon, or a member of the operating team, should come and personally speak to the family at the conclusion of surgery to inform them regarding how things went and what to expect in the short term. For any concerns, family members should feel free to check with the desk staff.

Elective brain surgery typically involves the patient being brought to the OR awake and oriented, followed by the placement of one or more IV lines if this had not already taken place in the preoperative or "holding" area. After the lines are placed, the patient breathes oxygen and anesthetic gases, is given IV sedation and, in this manner, is safely and comfortably put to sleep and intubated. **Intubation** involves placement of a breathing tube usually through the mouth and into the trachea for controlled ventilation during the procedure as the patient will be under deep anesthesia. A tube placed in this manner is referred to as an **endotracheal** (ET) **tube**. After this time, other lines are placed by the anesthesia team, such as an **intraarterial line** in the wrist artery for continuous blood pressure monitoring during the case, and possibly a deep IV line in the neck or upper chest called a "**central line**" for invasive monitoring of the patient's cardiovascular system. Thereafter, the neurosurgical team gets involved. The head is appropriately positioned for the surgery, and the body is well padded and secured to the OR table. The head is usually held in place during the surgery by a **pinion**, which is a metal clamp that has three points that enter into the skin of the scalp and are pressure-adjusted to make contact with the outer skull bone (**Figure 15**). The pinion, which keeps the head very still during surgery, is removed at the end of the procedure. The three pin holes are frequently filled with an antibiotic ointment after the pinion is removed, and the holes seal up on their own within 24 hours of surgery for the vast majority of patients. The pin sites typically pose no significant infection or cosmetic risk. They are very small and usually behind the hairline, although there may be one somewhere in the forehead which should also heal well.

After the patient is positioned, the scalp hair is shaved. The degree of the head shave varies from surgeon to surgeon. Many surgeons now prefer a relatively **minimal head shave**, namely, a 1-2 cm or half-of-one-inch wide strip of hair shaved in the appropriate location, typically behind the natural hairline (**Figure 16**). This is cosmetically appealing to most patients compared with a more extensive head shave, and there appears to be no proven downside to this, including no evidence of any increased infection if the usual "aseptic" measures are adhered to. Once the field is prepared with the appropriate antiseptic solutions and draped in a sterile manner, the OR scrub staff prepare the equipment around the field, and the surgery commences. The **incision** is made with a scalpel, and a scalp flap is turned and reflected to give good exposure of the cranial or skull bone and therefore the "**craniotomy site**". This site varies depending on the lesion, but most frequently involves the front and side of the head for **frontotemporal** and "**pterional**" **craniotomies**. There may be additional removal, followed by replacement at the end of the procedure, of the bones around the eye and/or cheek region as part of an "**orbitozygomatic**" (OZ) approach. Other frequent types of craniotomy for a lesion located at the back and under part of the brain near the brainstem, are those referred to as **suboccipital** and **retrosigmoid craniotomies**. The incision for the "frontotemporal crani" or one its variants goes from just in front of the ear, proceeds upwards and just behind the forehead hairline, and may swing slightly across the midline to the other side just behind the hairline (**Figure 16**). The incisions for the "suboccipital crani" and "retrosigmoid crani" are curved or linear ones located somewhere at the back of the head, depending on the location of the lesion (**Figure 17**).

Other specific craniotomies have incisions located differently. That is, a surgeon may use an incision almost anywhere in the scalp to gain the most direct access to an area of skull through which a **surgical window** can be made to get to the brain lesion or **surgical target**. The incision may be straight or **linear**, or shaped like a "C" or **horse shoe**, or gently curved like a **sutar**. When planning the **length and location of an incision**, a surgeon takes into consideration several factors including the site and size of the surgical target, the location of the nearest hairline, and the presence of any previous scalp incisions.

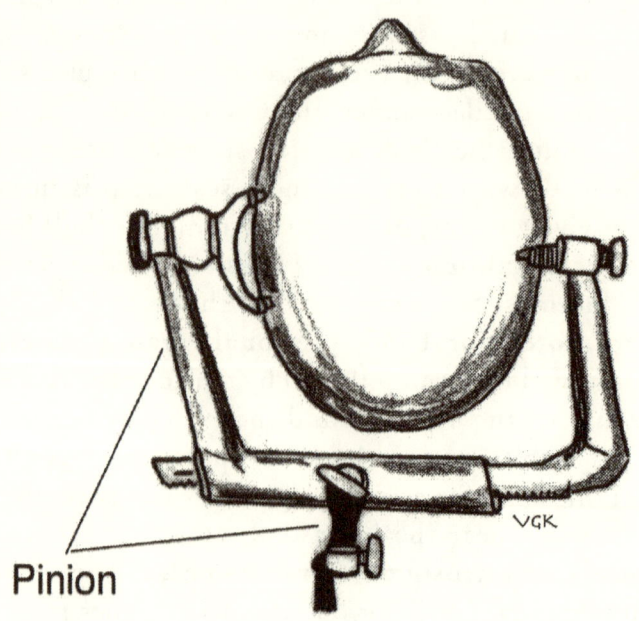

Figure 15. Pinion.

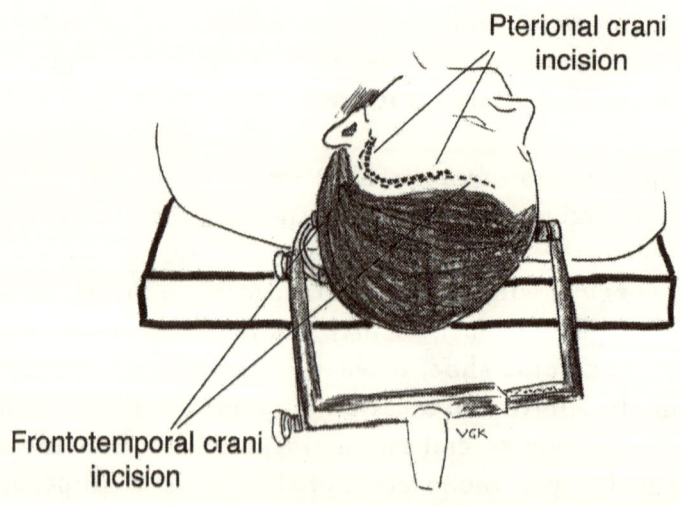

Figure 16. Minimal head shave and frontotemporal and pterional craniotomy incisions.

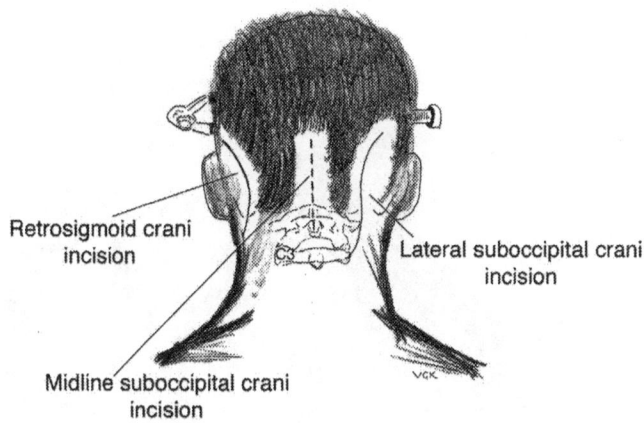

Retrosigmoid crani
incision

Lateral suboccipital crani
incision

Midline suboccipital crani
incision

Figure 17. Suboccipital and retrosigmoid craniotomy incisions.

After the scalp flap is turned, the exposed bone flap is removed using a high speed drill. Small "**burr**" **holes** are made in the skull and, with an appropriate attachment to seat the drill, the bone flap is removed (**Figure 18**). The dura is then exposed (**Figure 19**) and opened sharply with a scalpel and dural scissors. Once the dura is reflected out of the way, the brain surface is now seen (**Figure 20**).

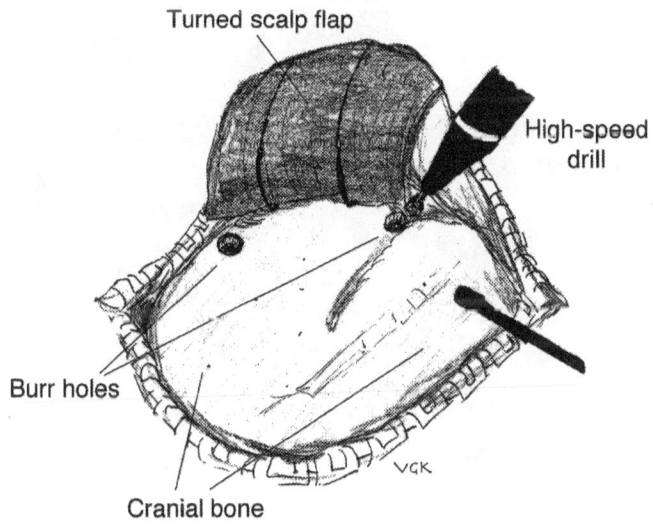

Turned scalp flap

High-speed
drill

Burr holes

Cranial bone

Figure 18. Scalp flap turned, cranium exposed, burr holes being drilled.

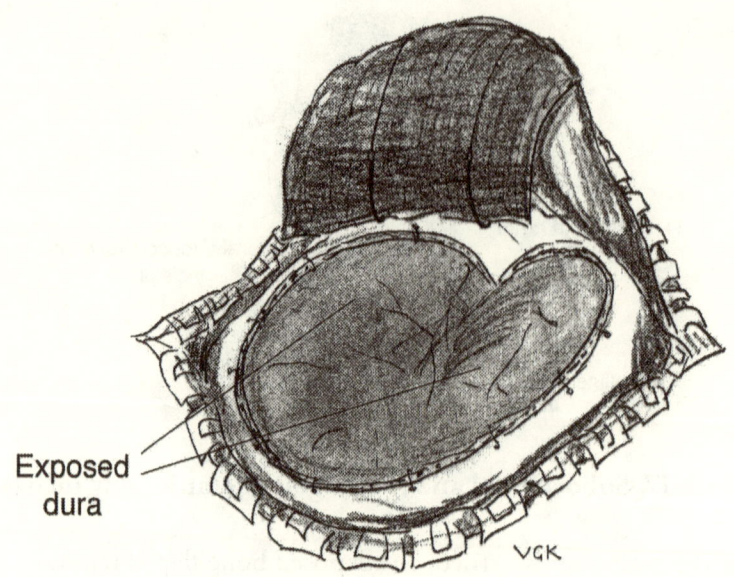

Exposed
dura

Figure 19. Bone flap removed and dura exposed.

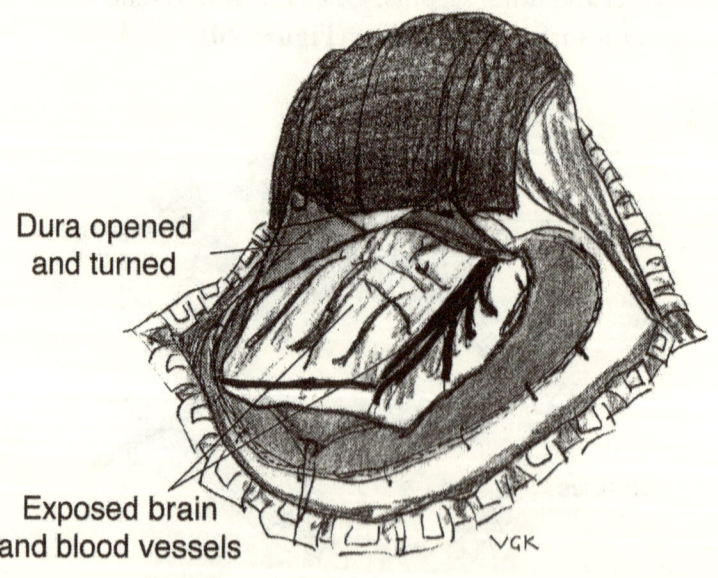

Dura opened
and turned

Exposed brain
and blood vessels

Figure 20. Dura opened and reflected, and brain surface exposed.

The **operating microscope** is brought into the field. The neurosurgeon then proceeds meticulously defining the nerve and vessel or **neurovascular structures** leading to and neighboring the brain lesion. The surgeon has available a wide variety of "microinstruments" to help in the dissection and removal or resection of the lesion, or its clipping if the lesion happens to be a brain aneurysm. At the conclusion of the procedure, when the field is dry, the dura is most often reapproximated with sutures. The bone flap is then replaced, typically affixed with **titanium miniplates and screws (Figure 21)**. It is restored so that a good cosmetic and structural result is obtained. The scalp is then closed with multiple layers of buried suture and either sutures or staples are used for the skin closure.

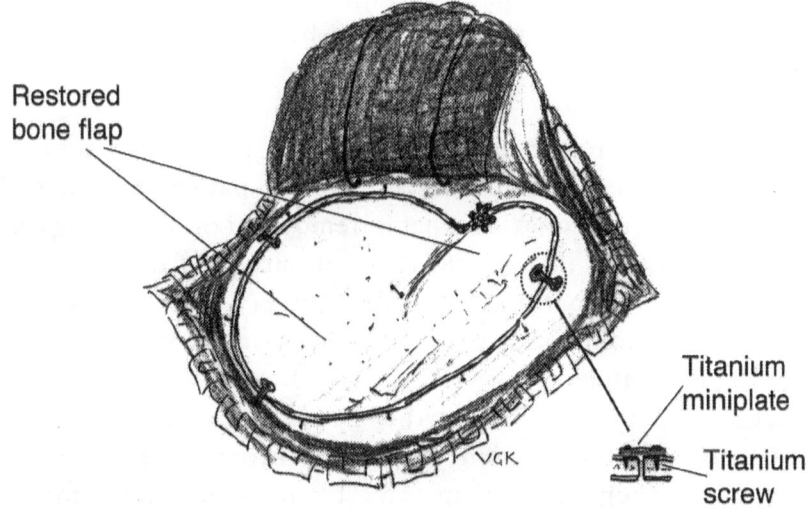

Restored
bone flap

Titanium
miniplate

Titanium
screw

Figure 21. Bone flap restored with titanium miniplates and screws.

Postoperatively, the patient will be transferred to the **ICU**. This is a fairly busy environment. Most have waiting areas for family members. Most have numerous medical and paramedical staff members. The rooms vary, some are one-patient only rooms, others accommodate two or more patients. There are many gadgets in each ICU room, with lots of lighted displays and sounds. Patients and family members should not be alarmed by these. The most obvious may be the monitor which displays the vital signs such as heart and breathing rate and rhythm, blood pressure, blood oxygen level, and so forth. There will be an IV line stand which holds the main IV fluid, and pain and other IV medications and, for some patients, a ventilator machine for the breathing tube. There may also be thin plastic drainage tubing coming from the patient's head or back to a nearby stand as part of the EVD or lumbar drain system (**Chapter 13**). The patient may have a **head wrap** on, which is like a white gauze turban with or without a fishnet outer wrap. In other words, a bandage that applies pressure around the head incision. There may be drainage tubing coming from this wrap, for a drain left under the scalp to drain blood that can accumulate underneath the incision edges. If the wrap and drain are present, they are generally removed the day after surgery. Some surgeons leave no head wrap, while others leave a head wrap on for 24-48 hours. The practice varies based on the surgeon's preference.

If a patient has returned to the ICU without an ET tube in, it means the anesthesiologist felt that the patient had met all requirements for **extubation**, that is, removal of the breathing tube following surgery. The patient therefore probably demonstrated to the anesthesia doctor at the end of surgery that he or she was able to follow commands by appropriately squeezing hands and wiggling toes, and was awake and strong enough to manage his or her own airway without further need for a tube. Note that a **breathing tube** causes some degree of throat irritation, and a patient may cough or spit up some blood-tinged saliva for the first few days after extubation. The patient may also have a dry or sore throat during this period, usually well treated with humidified air and throat lozenges. Such patients will usually be lucid or awake enough to talk and interact relatively well within a few hours of surgery. They still may be drowsy and in some pain. The drowsiness usually subsides on its own accord after the first night. The **head pain** subsides with appropriate pain medication. If the patient seems to be in pain that is not being appropriately controlled, the nursing and medical staff will alter the medications appropriately or ask for a "Pain Service" specialist to assist in the treatment. The vast majority of patients undergoing brain surgery do not experience significant incisional or operative pain after the first few days following the operation. However, they do experience some pain for the first 7-10 days after surgery, and usually this is well controlled with IV followed by oral narcotic medications over this period. The patient is asked to wean themselves off oral pain medications by 7-14 days as the pain gradually disappears.

The **ICU staff doctors** include a neurologist and/or an anesthesiologist with a special interest in critical care, and a neurosurgeon or neurosurgical resident or registrar. These doctors will regularly check on their ICU patients who will also be under the close supervision of the ICU nursing staff. The **nursing staff** will carry out and chart the regular neurological and vital observations of the patient, in addition to other "routine" but very important care of the patient including IV pain medication and fluid administration, patient positioning, pill and food administration and hygiene. Nurses will let the doctors know if there is any significant neurological change in the patient's state. Other **paramedical staff** may attend to ventilator management, urinary catheter management, and so forth, if the patient is still dependent on such equipment. The doctors and nurses generally make every attempt to **update families** daily. Note that at most centers, doctors round on their ICU patients at least twice daily. If patients or family members feel that there is not enough reasonable communication updating them or addressing their concerns, they should discuss this with the nursing or medical staff, or the ICU's nurse-manager.

If a patient returns to the ICU with an ET tube, the reasons may be multiple. It may be that the patient was in a poor neurological condition going into surgery. In such cases, the recovery will also be expected to be slow, and such patients may need more time before they are alert and strong enough to be safely extubated. Alternatively, the surgery may have been expectedly or unexpectedly complex, in which case the surgeon and anesthesiologist may favor keeping the patient intubated for the first night or so after surgery. Additionally, in surgery involving lesions near the brain stem, safe extubation may be hampered by swelling or damage of the lower brain stem pathways and nerves, some of which are very closely involved with respiration, speech and swallowing. For such patients, a longer period of intubation may be recommended or required to assist their breathing, and to prevent them from inhaling swallowed substances including saliva into their lungs, referred to as **aspiration**. The doctors should provide information regarding these matters and their reasoning for prolonged intubation (**Chapter 17**). Overall, the vast majority of brain surgery patients are successfully extubated at the conclusion of surgery.

Although events during the **early postoperative period**, that is, within the first 24-72 hours following surgery, vary according to the patient's neurological condition prior to surgery and the type of surgery, most **elective** neurosurgery patients are awake and talking on the night of the surgery, though they still may be drowsy. Most spend the first night in bed rest, with a Foley or urinary catheter and IV fluids and medications to help them along. Over the next day or two, many of these patients are encouraged to be sitting out of bed, and to begin eating. The earlier one is out of bed, the better it is for one's lungs which otherwise experience some degree of collapse and congestion in patients who for whatever reason are immobile or nonambulatory. Being **ambulatory** is also very helpful for the circulation, helping to prevent blood clots in the legs and lungs. In the day or few days after surgery, most neurosurgery patients should be expected to be walking again. Most will move from the ICU to a regular ward or "floor" bed after one or two nights, and many are dismissed from hospital after 3 or 4 nights. Many do not require any specific **physical therapy** (PT), but are rather encouraged to walk as much as possible. Climbing stairs is encouraged, as are eating a nutritious, well-balanced diet and gradually resuming regular activities including driving, sex, physical exercise, and work when their bodies tell them they are ready.

Hospital dismissal criteria for elective neurosurgery patients include being able to safely and independently walk, eat and excrete, in addition to having minimal, or at least well controlled, pain and a clean, dry and intact incision. At the time of a patient's dismissal, the medical team should provide the patient with a **written summary** of his or her stay and operation, and a telephone number for the patient to call if any neurological or wound or other concerns develop. The patient and family should be sure to have such **contact details** before leaving the hospital. Regarding the **postoperative followup visit**, a patient should check with the neurosurgeon or medical team regarding this. Many centers will automatically mail this appointment to the patient. The timing of the visit varies from patient to patient and from surgeon to surgeon. It cannot be overstated that appropriate followup for brain surgery patients is essential. Also, if a patient has **staples or sutures** in the incision at the time of dismissal, which is generally the case, someone needs to check on and remove them at the appropriate time, usually around **10-12 days after surgery**. This is referred to as a **wound check**. The patient's local doctor or nurse can remove these. Suture or staple removal is not a painful procedure. There may be slight tugging, but there should be no significant discomfort. Alternatively, the patient's surgeon or his or her assistant can remove these per the arrangements made at dismissal. In general, it takes anywhere between **3-12 weeks from the date of elective brain surgery for a patient to feel that he or she has significantly recovered to be able to resume a relatively normal life again.**

The early postoperative period for a neurosurgery patient operated on emergently, that is, under emergency or life-threatening conditions, may be different to the above. It heavily depends on the patient's neurological condition at the time of the hospital admission. First, such a patient may require more prolonged intubation or a more prolonged ICU stay. Second, such patients frequently take longer to mobilize as their brains have to heal from, say, blood being where it shouldn't be, or from herniation or other brain injury associated with their condition. As a result, they may take a few or several days, or even much longer, to be in a position to be safely moved out of bed, to finally walk, and be disconnected from all their drips, lines and tubes. They may have an EVD or lumbar drain, and require monitoring and treatment for the development of complications. A Physical Medicine and Rehabilitation (PMR) Service (**Chapter 20**) may be consulted to help in meeting the physical needs of such patients, with an aim to optimizing their overall recovery. There may be a need for only brief bedside PT. Alternatively, at some point during the hospital stay of an emergently treated neurosurgery patient, or an elective neurosurgery patient in whom a complication has arisen, it may be recommended that the patient undergo inpatient rehabilitation to further maximize the chance of an acceptable physical recovery (**Chapter 20**).

Finally, some words regarding **endoscopic brain surgery** or **neuroendoscopy**. Neurosurgery through an **endoscope**, which is a thin, tube-like telescope, is a form of **minimally invasive surgery** (MIS), or **"keyhole" surgery**. This means there is only a tiny skin incision, a small opening or burr hole or keyhole in the skull bone, and the procedure may be shorter in duration than for open surgery (**Figure 22**).

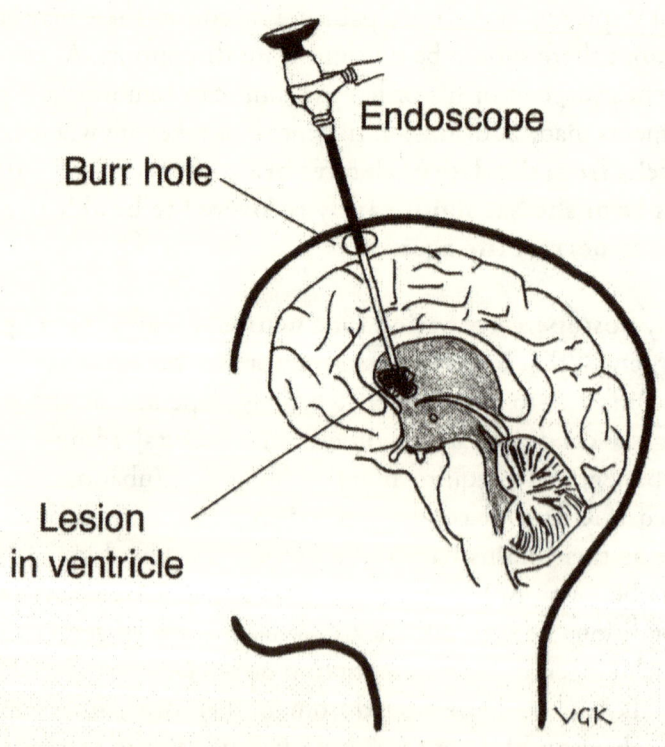

Figure 22. Keyhole or minimally invasive surgery: Neuroendoscopy.

MIS in the brain is carried out mainly 'for two reasons or "**indications**": (1) **Tumors** situated in the ventricles; and (2) **CSF diversion** in certain patients with obstruction of CSF drainage at the back of the brain's ventricular system, near a structure called the **cerebral aqueduct**. The former indication is referred to as an intraventricular tumor, the latter as an **endoscopic third ventriculostomy (ETV)**. For **intraventricular tumors**, the thin tubular endoscope is carefully advanced through the brain and into the ventricles. The neurosurgeon can watch the procedure in real-time on a television monitor because the endoscope has a light source and camera. The neurosurgeon maneuvers the endoscope through the ventricular system to the tumor, and using fine instruments deployed through the tube, can biopsy or remove the tumor in pieces. Sometimes there can be bleeding, and an EVD may need to be left to clear the CSF of blood after the procedure (**Chapter 13**). **During an ETV**, the endoscope is used to create a small hole in the floor of one of the ventricles known as the third ventricle. By doing so, CSF can be diverted by an alternative pathway, somewhat akin to an internal shunting procedure, except there is no tubing left behind. An ETV can not be carried out for all patients, and in some for whom it is carried out, the opening may close off, thereby requiring an actual shunt to be placed (**Chapter 13**). MIS is of course not without risk, but the risks are usually low (**Chapter 18**). The patient is asleep for the procedure, and many of the preoperative and postoperative issues mentioned earlier apply to MIS patients as well.

CHAPTER 13.

Drains, shunts, reservoirs, and needle biopsy with a head frame

There are several procedures carried out by neurosurgeons referred to as "**minor**" procedures. Of course, for a patient undergoing such a procedure, this may not at all be minor. Further, although these procedures are generally regarded as being of **low risk**, they are not of zero risk. The following procedures are carried out relatively frequently among neurosurgical patients as a group.

Drains

- **EVD**: An EVD allows CSF to be diverted temporarily from the ventricles to the outside world. Reasons for its placement include: (1) Hydrocephalus from any cause; (2) brain hemorrhage such as from an aneurysm or other lesion, particularly if the hemorrhage extends into the ventricles; (3) coma, particularly if associated with high ICP, in which case an EVD can be used to continually measure the ICP as well as to remove CSF periodically to lessen ICP; and (4) shunt infection, where the infected shunt is removed but CSF diversion is still required. An EVD consists of a **ventricular catheter**, which is a thin and flexible piece of tubing that will enter into the CSF-containing ventricle, in addition to tubing that will connect the ventricular end to a **measuring column and collection bag** kept at the patient's bedside (**Figure 23**). Placement of an EVD usually occurs in the ER or ICU. It is typically done using a local anesthetic to numb the skin, and after the area of the forehead scalp has been shaved and then "prepped" with antiseptic solution. Many patients undergoing EVD placement are semiconscious or unconscious owing to their underlying brain injury or disease process. Those who are conscious are usually administered some form of IV sedation to assist. A scalpel is used to make two small stab incisions in the numbed frontal scalp and a hand-held twist drill is used to make a small opening in the frontal bone through which the ventricular catheter is carefully threaded. Once CSF flow is detected through the catheter, it is sutured to the skin surface and its components hooked up. The whole procedure takes about 30 minutes from start to finish. EVD placement is generally regarded as a **low risk procedure**, however, there is a 1-2% chance of brain hemorrhage during placement and a 1-2% chance of infection. Here, infection may be a superficial wound infection or deeper infections such as ventriculitis or meningoencephalitis. To prevent this, IV antibiotic may be administered around the time of EVD placement, or the EVD tubing may itself be pre-impregnated with antibiotic. Periodically, CSF is sent off from EVDs to the laboratory for analysis. With time, the EVD is either "weaned" and removed, or converted to a lumbar drain or a shunt (see below).

- **Lumbar drain**: A lumbar drain is like a spinal tap or LP (**Chapter 6**), except that a thin and flexible piece of plastic tubing is intentionally left behind through the skin insertion point. The end of this tubing lies in the lumbar cistern. The tubing then runs on the surface of the back and is hooked up to a **collection bag** which is typically kept by the patient's bedside affixed to a mobile stand. A lumbar drain allows for **CSF diversion**, especially in cases where an EVD has been removed, and the patient may still be dependent on CSF removal for an anticipated few or several more days. Such drains can be placed in the setting of: (1) **Brain aneurysm rupture** in order to continue removing blood from the ventricles and cisterns;

(2) treatment of a **postoperative or posttraumatic CSF leak** from an incision or from the nose or ear, to allow pressure on the leak site to be reduced in order for it to heal; and (3) **preoperative preparation**, particularly for operations involving lesions located near the brainstem and cerebellum, where CSF removal from the drain will give good brain relaxation intraoperatively, and reduce the risk of CSF leak postoperatively. These drains are generally weaned and removed over three to four days after their placement. Lumbar drain insertion, like EVD placement, is a **low risk procedure**. There is a 1-2% chance of spinal hemorrhage or infection. The risk of hemorrhage is increased if the patient was recently on a **blood thinner** such as Plavix, or Coumadin/Warfarin. Once the drain is removed, there is a chance of a "**low pressure headache**" from ongoing CSF leak from the small pinhole in the spinal dura made during drain insertion. This can also occur following a regular LP, and can last several days. If it occurs, it is treated with bed rest for a few days, high oral fluid intake, and over-the-counter pain medications. If it persists for several days, an **epidural blood patch** may be recommended. This involves a second LP, this time injecting a certain volume of the patient's own blood through the needle to form a local clot that seals off the pinhole. Another complication of LP and lumbar drain placement is numbness and tingling in the legs. If it occurs, it should settle within hours to a few days. If worrisome, consult a physician. It is highly unlikely that there will be any permanent leg weakness or sensory problem from lumbar drain placement or LP.

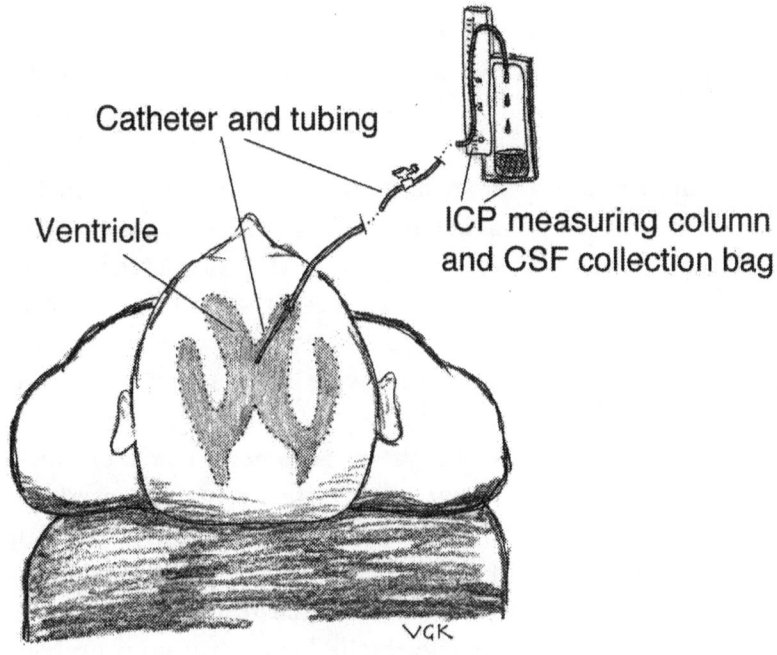

Catheter and tubing

Ventricle

ICP measuring column and CSF collection bag

VGK

Figure 23. EVD placement.

Shunts

A shunt is a piece of soft tubing that runs entirely under the skin surface from the ventricle or from the lumbar cistern to some other part of the body, most commonly the abdomen, but sometimes the lung or the neck. Shunts allow CSF to be continually diverted in patients who cannot absorb enough CSF for whatever reason. Shunts may be placed in patients who: (1) Are born with hydrocephalus; (2) **develop hydrocephalus** later in life following, say, brain aneurysm rupture, growth of an obstructive brain tumor, or some form of inflammation of the brain tissues such as in meningitis or ventriculitis; (3) cannot be successfully weaned from an EVD and/or lumbar drain; (4) have certain diseases such as NPH or BIHT. Shunt placement is carried out in the OR with the patient asleep. For the most common of shunt configurations referred to as the **ventriculoperitoneal (VP) shunt**, the shunt tubing runs from the ventricle to the abdomen's peritoneal space or **peritoneum**. The tubing runs in a fatty tunnel between the two locations. There will be a small, curved skin incision somewhere in the scalp overlying a small burr hole drilled in the adjacent skull bone, a second tiny straight incision somewhere behind the ear, and a slightly longer third straight incision somewhere in the abdomen. The tubing is tunneled by the surgeon between these three incisions (**Figure 24**). There is typically a bump felt near the scalp incision, which arises from placement of a **shunt valve** that regulates the flow of CSF. This should be expected to be felt in this location. The tubing can also be felt, but is otherwise invisible to the naked eye. The tubing and the valve are left in permanently unless a need for their removal arises, say, if the system becomes infected or blocked. Other shunt configurations include: (1) The **ventriculoatrial (VA) shunt** which runs from the brain's ventricle to the heart's right atrium through a small incision made in the neck to allow access to the internal jugular vein; (2) the **ventriculopleural shunt** which runs from the brain's ventricle to the lung's surrounding pleural cavity; and (3) the **lumboperitoneal shunt** which runs from the lumbar cistern to the abdomen's peritoneum. The concepts and tubing for these various shunt configurations are very similar. Shunt placement is generally regarded as a **low-risk procedure**. However, risks of shunt placement include a 10% chance of early or delayed infection requiring shunt hardware removal and replacement, a 10% chance of failure due to tubing disruption or blockage, and a 1-2% chance of hemorrhage in the brain or injury to the bowel during placement of a VP shunt. VA shunts have the added small risk of a significant heart rhythm disturbance, or arrhythmia, particularly at the time of VA shunt placement or very soon thereafter. **Symptoms and signs of shunt infection** usually manifest within the first few weeks of shunt placement, but may occur later. Symptoms can include unexplained fevers, redness along the shunt tubing site, headaches, nausea, vomiting, blurred vision, neck stiffness, increasing sleepiness, and sometimes increasing abdominal pain and tenderness.

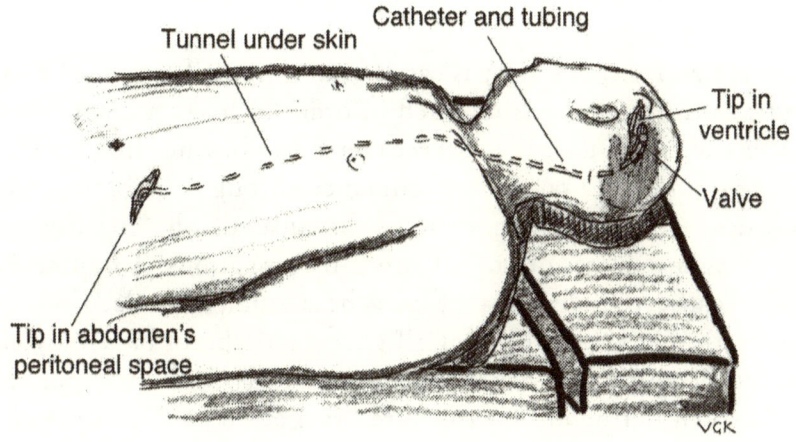

Figure 24. VP shunt placement.

Reservoirs

Reservoirs are small spaces enclosed by some form of plastic and buried under the skin surface. One end of a reservoir must end in a ventricle. The other end may be a dead end, as in the case of an **Ommaya reservoir**, or part of a shunt system's tubing. Reservoirs are typically placed in the OR with the patient asleep, but sometimes just sleepy, so that CSF can collect in them in order to allow future access to the inside of a shunt system, or to the ventricular system itself. CSF can be removed from reservoirs to: (1) Allow for its analysis in the setting of suspected shunt infection; or (2) immediately reduce abnormally elevated brain pressure. Removal of CSF from a reservoir is referred to as a **reservoir tap** and is usually done under local anesthetic using a very fine needle at the patient's bedside. In the case of an Ommaya reservoir, certain drugs such as chemotherapy and antibiotic agents can be injected through the reservoir directly into the ventricle in patients with certain brain tumors or infections. Placement of reservoirs is a very **low-risk procedure**, the main risks being a 1-2% chance of significant infection or hemorrhage during placement.

Stereotactic brain biopsy using a needle and head frame

A stereotactic brain biopsy is carried out if a small sample of brain and meningeal tissue is required in order to make a diagnosis of a specific brain disorder. **Stereotactic** implies needing specific image- and/or 3D coordinate guidance through the brain. Such biopsies are typically conducted because of the negative or "nondiagnostic" results of all other investigations (**Chapter 6**), and because the abnormality may be a small area deep within the brain. Unfortunately, not all stereotactic brain biopsies yield diagnostic results, but neurosurgeons will carry them out especially if they can define an **appropriate "target"** on the preoperative brain MRI. Usually, but not always, such a "preferred" target lights up abnormally on the MRI following administration of the IV contrast. If this target is successfully "hit" by the fine biopsy needle or probe, it is likely that some useful diagnostic tissue will be obtained. Many stereotactic brain biopsies involve the following, in this order:

- **Placement of a stereotactic head frame**: A head frame (**Chapter 14; Figure 25**) is an MRI-compatible metal structure that is affixed to the head with a minimum of **four pins** after the scalp has been prepared with antiseptic and numbed with local anesthetic. Head frame placement is usually done with the patient sleepy. As the pins are turned in and pushed deeper, there may be a pressure sensation which is uncomfortable. If there is a sharp painful sensation, the physician will administer more local anesthetic to the pin site. The scalp rapidly gets used to the pressure sensation, and the vast majority of patients tolerate head frame placement very well. The head frame allows for a very accurate 3D map of the patient's head and brain to be generated once the MRI is carried out. The head frame's accuracy and coordinate system generally rely on a suitable OR table device called a "receiving yolk" to which the head frame is subsequently attached, and an advanced computer and software system to carry out the calculations for the appropriate probe-target trajectory and depth.

- **Intubation of the patient**: The anesthesiologist will intubate the patient after the head frame is placed, and the patient is then taken to the MRI scanner asleep.
- **MRI head scanning with the head frame on**: The MRI scan will generate the images required to visualize the probe's trajectory prior to the procedure. Sometimes a CT scan is used instead.
- **Return to the OR asleep for needle biopsy**: The patient returns to the OR and, with the head frame on, is moved to the OR table. The head frame is attached to the receiving yolk. Several persons confirm the accuracy of the numbers and trajectory used for this procedure. The neurosurgeon makes a small incision in the scalp and carefully advances the biopsy needle along the chosen trajectory to the chosen depth. Usually a minimum of three small "core samples" are taken and sent to the OR pathologist for intraoperative confirmation that the tissue samples are indeed abnormal. The actual operating time for this procedure is usually only 30 minutes, however the procedure may take the good part of a day because of all of the steps involved, as indicated above.
- **Overnight ICU stay**: The patient is returned to the ICU, and observed overnight, particularly for signs of significant brain **bleeding or swelling**. The risks of these are small, in the order of 1-2%. The biopsy needle's small entry site in the scalp is usually closed with a self-dissolving suture, but this varies from surgeon to surgeon. The site may be covered by "skin glue" or a thin **Steristrip** or two. If present, Steristrips should be removed within one week of the procedure. Glue will dissolve with showering. Specifics of wound care should be discussed with the surgical team.
- **Await pathology and/or microbiology**: Samples that were taken during the biopsy are processed by the various laboratories, and a result is usually available within 48 hours of the procedure.
- **Dismissal with followup per a neurologist or neurosurgeon**: The patient is dismissed from the ICU either to his or her home or to a general ward, depending mostly on the patient's clinical state prior to the procedure. Followup will be arranged such that the patient meets with a physician after hospital dismissal to discuss the results of the biopsy and plan for appropriate treatment.

CHAPTER 14.

The radiosurgical procedure and early postoperative period

SRS involves the delivery of focused beams of radiation to a target such as a brain tumor. Although the word surgery is used, there is actually no skin incision, no open operation. SRS is really radiation therapy administered by a neurosurgeon or radiation oncologist with **surgical precision**. SRS has been used now for a few decades and in a few hundred-thousand patients. It is generally regarded as being safe and effective for a wide variety of brain conditions, including certain tumors and some AVMs. However, it is not without complications (**Chapter 18**). The reasons that SRS has not replaced open surgery as the gold standard for the majority of brain lesions include that SRS: (1) Typically **does not remove lesions** such as tumors, but rather tries to stop or arrest their growth by killing off their rapidly dividing cells; (2) is not as useful in the setting of large lesions, especially those **greater than 3 cm** in diameter, or those that are large and cystic or debris-filled; (3) does not alleviate the bad effects of lesions exerting **significant "mass"** within the brain, that is, lesions causing brain shift or impending herniation (**Chapter 5**); (4) is not effective for all lesions, as some are naturally **radiation-resistant**; and (5) can take **months or a few years** to work its effects on radiation-sensitive tumors or AVMs, respectively, and this timeframe may not be suitable for certain patients owing to the risks associated with such conditions during the time in which the patient is awaiting possible "cure". Having stated all of this, however, it cannot be denied that the availability of SRS has certainly played a **very beneficial role** in the treatment of many patients, especially those with: (1) Brain tumors, both primary and metastatic, **especially after surgical "debulking"**; and (2) lesions that are very deep in the brain, or spreading along the skull base.

There are several **different SRS systems** available to patients. Two very popular SRS systems discussed below are the Leksell Gammaknife® and the Accuray Cyberknife®. These systems are used in an **outpatient setting**, that is, half-day procedures with no hospital admission required. Although the systems can deliver all the radiation in one "sitting", sometimes the physician elects to have the lesion treated over a few sittings, something referred to as **hypofractionation** (HF). This may be safer for certain lesions near very critical structures, and HF may also be used for slightly larger lesions.

- **Gammaknife® (GK):** For the GK system, the patient is brought to the SRS suite, and local anesthetic is injected into 4 sites on the scalp, two at the front of the head and two at the back. Frequently, an oral or IV relaxing medication is administered, along with a dose of anti-inflammatory steroid. A relatively light-weight metallic **head frame** in the shape of a hollowed out cube is placed over the patient's head and the pins are advanced by wrench-tightening into the numbed scalp (**Figure 25**). If there is any pain during pin tightening, more local anesthetic is administered by the neurosurgeon. There may be some tight pressure as the pins are advanced to the skull's outer surface, but patients report that they adapt to this within minutes, and for the remainder of the procedure are comfortable. There is no need for intubation. After placement of the headframe, the patient is taken to the **MRI or CT scan** unit, and the scan is taken with the head frame incorporated into the scanned images. The images are verified by the neurosurgeon, and the patient returns awake to the **GK suite**. At this time, other members of the SRS team, including a radiation oncologist and a medical physicist, along with the neurosurgeon, use a sophisticated software program to plan the dose and configuration of the radiation to be administered. The brain images and head frame coordinates obtained from the head scan are used to create the safest and most precise or **conformal** dose plan. Once the plan is verified, the patient is placed on the GK table, which is like that of a CT or MRI scanner, and a hair-salon style helmet is placed over the headframe. This "**collimated**" **helmet** is metallic and has over 200 openings in it through which the fine radiation beams will pass. The patient, with helmet on, is advanced on the table into the doughnut-shaped radiation gantry of the GK unit, awake and freely able to talk with the GK staff, and at the same time be monitored by them throughout the procedure. The radiation "shots" are administered in short stages, and the patient's head position frequently needs to be changed. The radiation delivery itself typically takes a few hours to complete. At the end of the procedure, the patient is observed briefly and then dismissed to home. It is recommended that the patient have someone accompany them in order to safely transport the patient home at the end of the day. Appropriate followup should be discussed and/or arranged by the surgeon before the patient leaves the unit.

- **Cyberknife® (CK):** For the CK system, there are no pins, no head frame, and no helmet. There is no need for any anesthesia or "premedication" except for a dose of steroid per the physician's preference. The **CK suite** includes a radiation device called a mini-linear accelerator or **Linac** to deliver the radiation, and this is mounted on a **computer-controlled robotic arm (Figure 26)**. Uniquely, the system uses real-time **image guidance technology** to monitor the patient's breathing movements and any head or torso movements, and can adjust or fine-tune the Linac's direction accordingly, in order to maintain its safety and accuracy. Instead of an invasive head frame, the CK system uses a flexible breathe-through mesh **face mask** and/or **torso frame** to keep the patient as still as possible during the procedure. The CK system also has the advantage of being able to be used throughout the body, that is, for tumors and other lesions in the spine, chest, abdomen, pelvis, and so forth. Once the radiation plan is made with the help of the CT or MRI scan, the radiation delivery takes place over a period of 60-90 minutes. No alteration of the patient's position is required to carry out the delivery. The patient is observed briefly, and then dismissed to home. Again, followup should have been arranged.

Complications of SRS are discussed elsewhere (Chapter 18). Interestingly, advocates of the GK system claim that the headframe makes the targeting more accurate compared with the CK system. On the other hand, advocates of the CK system claim that it is as accurate as the GK system, avoids placement of a headframe and helmet, and can be used for different body regions. Overall, many neurosurgeons feel that **these two excellent systems are very comparable for the purpose of focused brain radiation delivery.**

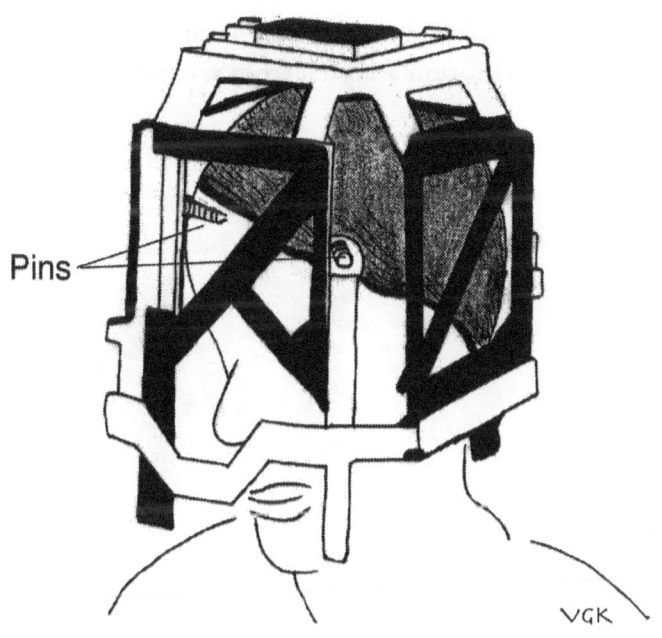

Figure 25. Gammaknife® head frame for accurate targeting.

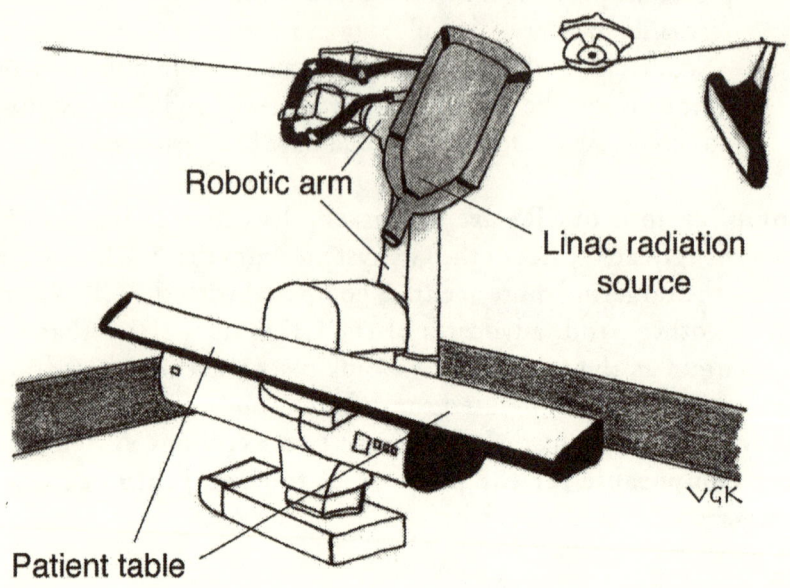

Robotic arm

Linac radiation source

Patient table

Figure 26. Cyberknife® robotic arm for accurate Linac radiation targeting. Illustration adapted from www.accuray.com.

CHAPTER 15.

The endovascular surgical procedure and early postoperative period

Just as for the perioperative period, the **periinterventional period** refers to the few days before and after endovascular treatment of the lesion. The **endovascular surgeon** will meet with the patient to discuss the benefits, risks, alternatives, team approach and technical and recovery aspects of endovascular surgery. An **anesthesiologist** may meet with the patient to make sure the patient is medically cleared for the procedure, even if it is not an open surgical one and even if the patient is not required to be in deep anesthesia for the procedure. For some brain lesions being treated with microcoils and/ or stents, the endovascular surgeon may make a recommendation for the patient to be placed on some form of **blood thinner** such as Plavix for the procedure. The rationale for this is that having a blood thinner on board prior to the placement of microcoils and/or a stent will prevent the arteries around the lesion from suddenly blocking off or thrombosing, which can cause a stroke. Thrombosis happens because microcoils and stents are **intrinsically thrombogenic** in that they slow blood flow around them enough to cause blood to clot. The endovascular surgeon will tell a patient if he or she wants the patient to be "loaded" with a blood thinner before the procedure. The load, if recommended, is usually administered as an oral medication the night before the procedure, but sometimes is administered as an oral or IV medication at the very time of the procedure.

The **preinterventional period** involves a patient eating and drinking nothing from midnight before the morning of the procedure, and checking with his or her doctor beforehand regarding taking any medications. Most endovascular surgeons will want to carry out such procedures earlier in the day rather than later, and after reporting to the patient registration area of the hospital at the specified time, the patient will be directed to the angiography suite in which the procedure will be carried out.

Generally, endovascular treatment is free of pain. There may or may not be a requirement for deep or **general anesthesia**, depending on the brain condition, the patient, and the type of endovascular treatment. If no deep anesthesia is required, it is likely that a **modified attended anesthesia** routine will be used, where oxygen is administered via face mask or nasal cannula and mild IV sedating medications used to make the patient drowsy and settled but still somewhat cooperative. Just as for cerebral angiography (**Figure 14**), local anesthetic is administered at the catheter entry site typically in the groin region and the thin **catheter tubing** is advanced painlessly through the aorta and into the arteries of the neck and brain. When the **contrast dye** is injected into the patient's circulation through the catheter itself, there may be a warm rushing sensation felt by the patient, but there should be no other significant discomfort. As the dye is injected, the X-ray machines are operative, rapidly taking multiple X-rays and forming a roadmap of the patient's brain circulation. The lesion is identified, and the microcoil or stent or glue is introduced or **deployed** through the catheter into the lesion (**Figure 27**). The lesion is then shut down or occluded, hopefully completely and without complication. The devices are withdrawn and manual pressure is held over the femoral "puncture" site for about 20-30 minutes to allow a suitable clot to form. An arterial closing device may be used instead. The endovascular procedure itself may take anywhere between 1-3 hours. Additional time may be taken for appropriate anesthesia and post-procedural recovery. The patient may be kept flat in bed for about 4-6 hours after the catheter is removed to allow the femoral clot to form, so that no hemorrhage occurs at or from this site. A hemorrhage or **hematoma** at this site is usually marked by an expanding and often painful thigh clot. The patient should report this to the nursing staff who, in any case, should be checking for its occurrence regularly after the patient returns to Recovery and then the ICU area.

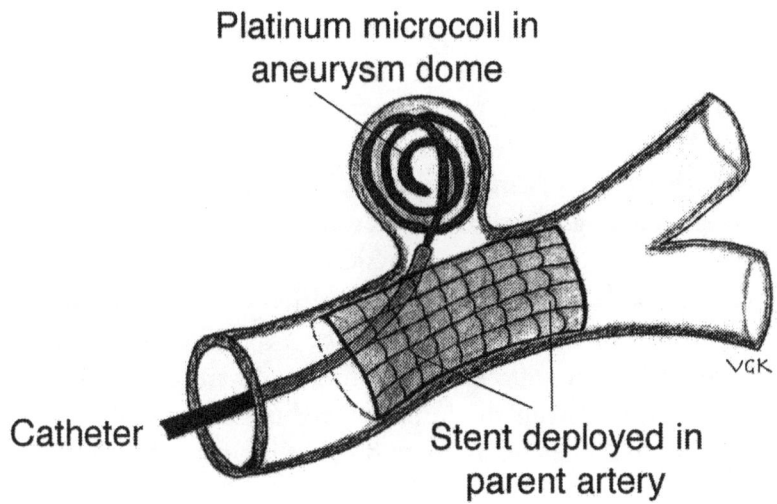

Platinum microcoil in
aneurysm dome

Catheter

Stent deployed in
parent artery

Figure 27. Endovascular coiling and stenting.

Most endovascularly treated patients are taken to the ICU for one night. Many are dismissed from the ICU directly to home the next morning. Exceptions to early dismissal include: (1) A **ruptured aneurysm patient**, whose postprocedural care may be complex; (2) a patient who suffered a **complication** during the endovascular procedure; and (3) a patient whose endovascular procedure was the first of a **multi-stage treatment plan** where, say, the second stage involves open surgery a day or two after the first stage. For most patients who have undergone uncomplicated elective endovascular treatment, the night of the procedure is generally unremarkable. They should be awake, talking and appropriately interactive early after the procedure, and are frequently encouraged to get out of bed to a chair after a brief period of postprocedural bed rest. There is very little by way of pain. The two **pain issues** are some degree of **headache**, which is common after coiling of aneurysms particularly in the posterior circulation, and the occurrence of minor thigh aching pain from the puncture site. The endovascular surgeon should make recommendations regarding the treatment of the headache, which usually involves oral medications for a few days. This dull or throbbing headache, if it occurs at all, usually subsides within a few days, and is not like the severe thunderclap headache of aneurysmal rupture. If the latter happens at any time after the procedure, the patient should seek medical attention immediately. Sometimes higher doses of a nonsteroidal anti-inflammatory medication such as Motrin, Advil, or ibuprofen can be used regularly for a few days till the headache subsides, but a patient should check with the endovascular surgeon first. On the day of dismissal, usually the day after the procedure, patients should be given clear **contact and followup instructions**. If not, they should check with their physician and nursing care givers. It is vital that the patient returns for followup after endovascular treatment of his or her lesion, because there may be a significant chance of the lesion's recurrence or regrowth depending on its size and/or its degree of obliteration following the initial procedure. The timing of future angiograms should be communicated to the patient before leaving the hospital.

CHAPTER 16.
Wound issues

Wound healing is a very important aspect of surgery and postoperative recovery. It can be **impaired** by **preexisting medical problems** such as diabetes mellitus, poor nutrition, poor levels of activity, **smoking**, and chronic use of steroids or nonsteroidal anti-inflammatory medications such as ibuprofen and aspirin. Other things that can lead to wound problems include **eyeglass frames** continually rubbing over the incision or a patient **scratching** the incision. Conversely, a good balanced diet, regular walking, and multivitamins are likely to be of benefit. For eyeglass wearers undergoing frontotemporal craniotomy, it is recommend that a soft padded piece of gauze taped to the glasses' frame be used as a buffer between the underlying incision and the plastic or metal frame near the ear. This padding should be worn till a few days after the sutures or staples are removed, that is, for a period of around two weeks. If soiled or damp, the padding should be changed as needed during this time.

Surgical wounds should be treated with respect. Many surgeons feel that **showering** is okay some time the day after surgery. The wound does not need to be covered during showering, however it is recommended that no direct shower spray be applied to the incision. It is acceptable for water to run over the incision. At the end of the shower, the incision should be gently dabbed dry, not rubbed or abraded. A patient should avoid shampooing the hair for the first 48 hours after surgery. Thereafter, a baby shampoo can be used everywhere except directly on the incision. Generally, one should not apply creams, oils or ointments to the incision. It is best to let the incision air dry. Some neurosurgeons recommend not to take a tub or spa bath or enter a swimming pool for the first 2-3 weeks after surgery, as dampness may breed infection. However, this recommendation varies between surgeons, so a patient should check with his or her surgeon first. A few days to a week after the staples or sutures have been removed, it is okay to commence normal showering, bathing and shampooing as long as the incision looks fine. It takes several weeks to a few months for the deep tissues to heal well. Any signs of wound infection, as detailed below, should be reported to the doctor at once. **Sutures and staples** come out somewhere between 10-12 days after surgery. If a subcuticular closure was carried out where no sutures were left on the skin surface but rather buried under the skin, then **Steristrips**, which are butterfly-like stickies, may have been applied to the skin surface instead. These need to come off after a shower by 7 days following surgery. Leaving these strips on longer than 7 days increases the buildup of grime and the chance of infection. Sometimes, a skin glue is used and this should dissolve within a few days of showering. Suture and staple removal can be carried out by the patient's local nurse or doctor, or by the neurosurgeon or his or her assistant. Although there may be some gentle tugging, suture or staple removal is not painful and there is no injection. Some neurosurgeons recommend a period of 24 hours shower-free following suture or staple removal so the tiny holes can seal up.

There are a number of issues that may arise regarding the incision or the operative site. Each of these is worth considering one-by-one:

- **Wound infection**: Despite the best efforts of neurosurgeons and OR personnel, and attempts to adhere to strict aseptic technique intraoperatively, approximately 1-2 in every 100 craniotomy patients get a wound infection. That is, there is a **1-2% infection rate**. There is a 1% chance of wound infection at the groin puncture site for angiography or coiling. Many of these infections are **superficial**, and require only a brief course of oral antibiotic therapy. Others, however, are **deep**, and require reopening of the incision, cleansing of the infected tissue, debridement of the infected skin edges and, where applicable, possibly removal of the bone flap, which may need to be discarded. In such cases, which are rare, the bone flap may eventually be replaced months later with a synthetic bone substitute or a titanium mesh. This is known as a **cranioplasty**. Wound infections generally become obvious about **10-14 days after surgery**. A small amount of redness and mild swelling near the incision itself is normal early after open surgery, however, this should have subsided by 5-6 days postoperatively. At 10-14 days after surgery, if the wound is getting more red, swollen or "boggy", and tender, or if it begins to drain blood-stained fluid, these are signs that the patient needs to seek medical attention at once. Unexplained fevers associated with headache, nausea and vomiting, or neck stiffness or confusion are signs that a deep infection may be involving the brain or its coverings. Patients with suspected wound infections should be examined by their local doctor or neurosurgeon, and the appropriate action taken. The doctor can follow a patient's healing from a wound infection clinically by bedside examination and certain blood tests and radiologically via a head CT scan. Most wound infections resolve with the appropriate management. Those few patients requiring bone flap removal generally have good outcomes after a cranioplasty is carried out to restore cosmetic and structural integrity in the operated region. During the time the bone flap is removed, no full-time helmet is required for most adults, rather, just general precautions against falls and head injuries once the patient returns home, awaiting future cranioplasty. The patient should avoid bike riding, roller blading, and contact sports during the period that the bone flap is removed, and for 2 months following cranioplasty, or as advised by the surgeon.

- **CSF leak**: Leakage of clear tear-like fluid from an **incision** or other site following brain surgery is uncommon, but something that needs to be reported to the doctor should it occur. Other sites that CSF may leak from, depending on the site of surgery, include the ear, an event known as **otorrhea**, or the nose, an event known as **rhinorrhea**. CSF rhinorrhea may manifest as a continuous salty taste down the back of the throat, or tear-like fluid dripping like a tap from the nose. CSF leaks from incisions can be treated by oversewing the wound in the Office or ER under local anesthetic, with recheck in an outpatient setting. Alternatively, placement of a lumbar drain for a few days and a pressure head wrap with observation in a hospital in-patient setting may be recommended. It is very rare for a patient to require surgery specifically for a postoperative CSF leak, in this case exploration and revision of the wound, if there is no hydrocephalus causing the leak. Here, **hydrocephalus** causes an increase in pressure within the brain, and forces CSF out a path of least resistance, such as a fresh incision or a previous EVD site. If there is delayed hydrocephalus, which is uncommon but can occur in, say, ruptured aneurysm or brain tumor patients, shunt placement is usually recommended.

- **Swelling**: It is normal to experience some swelling in the incision area following surgery. Sometimes the swelling is dramatic, and can even cause the eye on the same side of the surgery to be swollen shut for a few or several days. There may be bruising of the affected eye depending on the type of craniotomy, and this may persist for several weeks before subsiding. This is particularly common in **OZ craniotomies**. For swelling in the wound area, icepacks and walking around can be helpful. Except for patients undergoing OZ craniotomies in whom eye swelling is expected to last in the order of weeks, if swelling around the face and incision has not begun to subside by 3-5 days after neurosurgery, the patient should contact his or her doctor. Sometimes CSF or dissolving blood clot fluid can collect under the scalp, and usually this resolves by reabsorbing on its own after a few to several days. However, if the collection under the scalp enlarges, it may be a sign that the patient has some degree of hydrocephalus, especially in the case of a ruptured aneurysm or incompletely removed tumor. A CT scan of the head should be obtained. This may also rule out infection of the underlying deep scalp and skull bone as a cause of delayed swelling in a wound.

• **Cosmetic issues**: The vast majority of craniotomy wounds heal very well, and are generally invisible as most lie behind the hairline. However, some craniotomies can be "complicated" by cosmetic issues. For example, there may be some loss of muscle bulk, referred to as **atrophy**, in the **temporalis muscle**. This is a chewing muscle at the side of the head in the "temple" or temporal region, just in front of and above the ear. The temporalis muscle is taken down, and at the end of the procedure reattached, during a frontotemporal or "pterional" craniotomy. Note that in a mini-OZ craniotomy, carried out by some neurosurgeons for certain lesions, there is only a minimal cut in the muscle, thereby making temporalis muscle atrophy less likely to occur. Another cosmetic issue may be that the **bone flap** may **settle** such that a ridge is seen or felt, or a titanium miniplate or screw head is felt. When weighing up survival from a significant brain disorder versus these cosmetic issues, patients and physicians alike tend to agree that these cosmetic nuisances are part and parcel of surgery.

• **Pain, numbness and dysesthesia**: There will be **pain** after surgery, because tissues were incised in order to carry out the operation. For most patients, the pain is well controlled with IV medications early after surgery, converted to oral pain medications soon thereafter. By 2-4 days, the pain is substantially better for most patients, and almost resolved by 7-10 days. Pain medications are then weaned. The **pain threshold** for each patient varies, but by far the majority are pain free somewhere within 2 weeks. Persistent pain is uncommon and should be reported to the doctor. Many patients report some form of isolated **numbness** or a strange feeling referred to as "**dysesthesia**" around some part of the incision. This is likely due to cutting of small sensory nerves in the incision site. This tends to resolve in weeks to months, however at times it may persist. There is generally no treatment sought or offered for this, as again, weighing this against the serious nature of many brain conditions puts things in perspective for patients and doctors alike. Additionally, some patients report discomfort with **chewing**, or incomplete **mouth opening**. This is more commonly reported following a frontotemporal or full-OZ craniotomy in which the temporalis muscle is incised early in the operation. This generally resolves as the incision heals, but it may take several days to several weeks. **PT for the jaw** is recommended for those rare patients with significant or persistent symptoms. Finally, some patients undergoing a craniotomy report symptoms such as "fluid in the ear" or "ear fullness" or a "crackling sound". These **ear symptoms** typically settle within days to weeks. If fluid is dripping from the ear, a patient should report this to his or her doctor.

CHAPTER 17.

Issues concerning comatose and critically ill patients

A comatose patient is one who is generally regarded as exhibiting little or no spontaneous self-generated activity, apart from breathing, and being unresponsive or poorly responsive to the outside world. Coma can arise in the setting of an advanced brain tumor, severe TBI, brain hemorrhage, and so forth. The care of a comatose patient is complex. Significant and meaningful recovery may indeed be delayed by weeks to months, and at times there may be no meaningful recovery. In the best interests of comatose patients, the medical team generally tends to be aggressive with the care of such patients, whenever such a stance is appropriate and potentially beneficial. The level of care offered may evolve according to the progress of the patient as time passes. It is expected that any significant change in the level of care offered to a patient will only be set in place after a thorough and informed discussion between the physician and the patient's family members is undertaken, reaching a mutually acceptable "consensus".

There are many aspects of a comatose patient's care worth considering:

- **Advance directive** (AD): An AD is some form of legal document such as a **Living Will** or a special hospital AD form signed and dated by a patient, licensed health care provider and a witness. Alternatively, it may be a **Health Care Power of**

Attorney (POA) Plan. An AD provides some direction to health care workers regarding the patient's desired level of care should certain circumstances arise making the patient unable to communicate or provide health care directives. Such situations include coma or significant cognitive impairment following admission, from any cause. It is important for a patient to **plan ahead** by making an AD and discussing it with his or her spouse and other family members and doctor. In considering the following, a patient should be sure to obtain the up-to-date and location-specific recommendations that apply to him or her self. What follows are general points. First, an AD can be changed or revoked by the patient at any time. The cognitively unimpaired patient has the capacity and right to decide regarding the type of treatment he or she may wish if certain critical circumstances arise. Life-sustaining treatments he or she should consider include mechanical ventilation, dialysis, blood transfusion, antibiotic therapy, and artificial nutrition and hydration therapies. Second, ADs may include a status order such as "**do-not-resuscitate**" (**DNR**) or "**do-not-intubate**" (**DNI**) in the event of cardiorespiratory arrest, that is, when heart and/or lung function ceases, or if other major clinical decline occurs in a patient rendering him or her critically ill and unable to appropriately provide directives at that time. Note that a physician directly involved in a patient's care can write a DNR status for a comatose or seriously ill and severely incapacitated patient but this should be discussed with family and colleagues and the appropriate consensus reached. Third, a Living Will should clearly state the circumstances and details of health care that a patient does or does not wish to have. This document should be signed and dated by the patient and a notary. Here, an appropriate notary is an independent person who is not a beneficiary of the patient's Will, and not his or her health care provider, POA, guardian, surrogate or next of kin. A Health Care POA document should be signed and dated in a similar manner. Finally, when considering ADs, the patient's wishes and best interests should always be put first. To the best of their abilities, physicians and family should try to determine what the patient would desire if he or she was able to make ongoing care decisions. The preferences of the patient should prevail.

- **Chest percussion therapy** (CPT): This is provided by one or more respiratory therapists, nurses, and also certain modern ICU beds themselves. It involves vibrating or clapping on a patient's chest in order to break up secretions that can build up after prolonged periods in the supine or lying down position encountered in comatose patients. It is an important part of preventing or minimizing collapse in the lungs referred to as **atelectasis**, which can be a breeding ground for inflammation and/or infection of the lungs, that is, **pneumonitis** or **pneumonia**.

- **Feeding and Nutrition**: If a patient is comatose, it goes without saying that he or she will not be able to voluntarily eat. As a result, a **feeding tube**, which is a thin and soft plastic tube, may be passed by a physician or nurse from the nose of a patient into the patient's stomach for feeding and oral medication administration purposes. After a significant period of time, such as a few weeks, this tube may be converted by a general surgeon or gastroenterologist to a "**PEG**" or "**PEJ**". This is a **percutaneous gastrostomy or jejunostomy**, respectively, which is essentially a tube directly inserted from the abdominal skin surface into the stomach or adjacent small intestine for long-term feeding purposes. The type of feeding formula provided through either a feeding tube or a PEG or PEJ varies according to the hospital's practices and recommendations of the hospital Nutrition Service.

- **Ventilation and airway support**: A comatose patient is unable to safely support their own airway and may be unable to generate enough airway pressures and volumes to effectively breathe. In such circumstances, they are placed on mechanical ventilators or breathing machines until they reach a point at which they no longer require the apparatus, or use of the apparatus is discontinued. In order to keep the airway of a comatose patient open, an ET tube is used. If still needed after about one week, this may be converted over to a **tracheostomy** tube, or "trache". A tracheostomy is a very short-tube airway inserted directly through the throat into the windpipe. It is placed in order to prevent pressure-related injury from an ET tube to the patient's airway tissue. In order to talk with a tracheostomy tube, the tube needs to be manually "capped" at the throat surface. With recovery, the tracheostomy can be removed and the throat opening sutured close.

- **Repositioning and skin care**: Changing a comatose patient's body position and vigilant monitoring of the patient's skin for signs of pressure-related injury are essential in preventing skin breakdown and infection. Such infection can even spread to the blood stream, an event referred to as wound-related **sepsis**. Nurses and physical therapists (PTs) are particularly attentive to this. Should **pressure-sores** develop, they are treatable, but perhaps the best treatment is prevention. Sometimes treatment requires the input of a skin care nurse specialist or a plastic surgeon.

- **Toileting and hygiene**: A comatose patient typically still has bowel and bladder function. The IV fluids are eventually excreted by the kidneys and out through the urethra, into a urinary or **Foley catheter** tube. The catheter is periodically changed to prevent infection, while urine samples are periodically sent to the laboratory to evaluate for signs of infection. Regarding the passage of feces in comatose patients, although defecation may be less frequent, this may occur directly onto bed sheets. Clothing and linen are typically immediately changed by the nursing staff to prevent infection and maintain optimal patient health and hygiene. Further, regular bed baths, including sponge or cloth baths in addition to hair, skin and oral hygiene are provided by nursing and paramedical staff. All of these are important in, among other things, maintaining the dignity of comatose patients.

- **Bedside PT**: This is discussed in detail elsewhere (**Chapter 20**).

- **Prevention of deep venous thrombosis** (DVT) **and pulmonary embolism** (PE): A **deep venous thrombus** is a blood clot that develops usually in a deep or major leg vein, but sometimes also in a deep arm vein. Such clots may develop because that limb is not working normally, spending most of the time lying dormant in a comatose patient, despite the efforts of nursing staff and PTs. DVT usually presents with limb swelling in comatose patients, while awake patients frequently report limb aching discomfort. A limb ultrasound usually confirms the presence of the clot. The major risk of DVT is migration of clot fragments into the circulation and lodging in the lung. This event is referred to as **pulmonary embolism** (PE), which can be fatal. Treatment options that may be required in the setting of new DVT/PE include IV blood thinners if deemed safe enough to use or if there is no effective alternative to their use, and placement of a **vena cava filter**. Such a filter is a small umbrella that collects clot material before it can reach the heart and lungs. To **prevent DVT/PE** in the first place, medical teams usually use thigh or knee-high **thromboembolic disease** (TED) **stockings/hose** in bedbound patients, and **sequential compression devices** (SCDs). The latter are automatically reinflating devices that squeeze the calf muscles to circulate blood in this region, thereby attempting to minimize hemostasis or slowed blood circulation that otherwise promotes the occurrence of DVT. Also, many doctors will use **subcutaneous** (SQ) **shots** of low dose blood thinners, such as SQ heparin or Fragmin or Lovenox, or some equivalent. Early mobilization of a patient is also very helpful, but hard to do if the patient is comatose.

- **CSF drainage**: Matters related to EVD and lumbar drain placement have been discussed in detail elsewhere (**Chapter 13**).
- **Disposition**: This refers to the appropriate "placement" for comatose patients. It generally refers to their place in an ICU, as their vital functions cannot be adequately monitored and supported in any other setting. However, for comatose patients in whom ICU status is no longer deemed effective or appropriate and therefore withdrawn after appropriate discussions, disposition may then be a hospital ward, or a hospice or nursing home facility, or home. This depends on the medical condition of the patient and other factors, including logistic factors such as bed availability and the family's resources. Disposition may be guided by the medical condition of the patient, ADs of the patient, and family members' wishes, with the aid of nursing staff and a Social Worker.

- **Withdrawal of support** (WOS): WOS issues are very
  important considerations in those patients who are deemed
  by physicians and family members alike as being in so
  poor a neurological condition that a meaningful recovery
  is essentially not likely to occur. WOS must take into
  consideration the patient's documented or perceived
  expectations under these conditions. WOS generally means
  that all life-sustaining treatments, investigations, and
  supportive therapies will cease, including ventilator and
  supplemental oxygen support, blood and imaging tests, IV
  hydration, all medications other than pain medications,
  and all nutrition. In the place of these, physicians will
  usually prescribe "**comfort care**" measures, including
  only a regular dose of SQ or IV pain medication such as
  Morphine or Fentanyl and humidified air for a patient's
  breathing comfort. The goals of a WOS scenario are to
  continue to relieve pain and suffering and to provide and
  promote dignity in the patient's last few hours or days. A
  WOS scenario may forseeably hasten death as opposed
  to prolonging a patient's "life" in a **persistent vegetative
  state**. Physicians and family members alike must feel that
  the WOS status is appropriate, with adequate levels of
  informed communication between physicians and family
  members. Sometimes there arises a need for institutional,
  that is, hospital-based, or judicial, that is, legal body-based,
  intervention. This may occur if there is no significant
  family member or surrogate available, or if a dispute occurs
  among significant family members in the absence of ADs,
  or if a doctor feels that there is a conflict between a family's
  interests and a patient's best interests in absence of an
  AD. A **hospital Ethics Service Consultation** or **Ethics
  Committee** may be asked to provide input, but this is
  generally not legally binding. Rather, it serves more of an
  advisory role. Such a committee or Service may consist
  of an independent doctor, nurse, Justice of the Peace or
  attorney, a hospital administrator, a social worker, and a
  chaplain.

- **Caring for the caregiver**: Although last in this chapter, it is by no means least. Being diagnosed with and treated for a brain condition is not only extremely stressful for the patient, but also stressful for the loved ones of the patient. Broken sleep, continuous worrying, and often the alien environment and unfamiliar faces of a large hospital can take their toll on the physical and emotional health of the patient's loved ones. That is why it is important to note that, to the best of their ability, loved ones should maintain regular and healthy rest and nutrition practices. It should be remembered that a patient's healing is closely related to the support of his or her family and social network. Therefore, the ongoing health and wellbeing of a patient's loved ones are important parts of the overall healing and recovery equation.

CHAPTER 18.

Complications of treatment

No treatment option is free of risk of complications. The risk of complications is dependent on many factors including:

- **The size and location of the lesion**: As a rule of thumb, larger lesions and lesions located in the deep parts of the brain, or in the brain stem carry higher treatment-related risks.
- **How the lesion presented at the time of treatment**: For example, a patient with a metastatic brain tumor presenting with a large brain hemorrhage within the tumor bed may have a lower chance of a good outcome. The same can be said for a patient with a brain aneurysm who presents following rupture of the aneurysm. These outcomes are more dependent on the clinical condition of the patient prior to treatment, rather than the treatment itself.
- **The type of treatment offered**: For a certain lesion in a certain patient, it may be deemed by the physician to be safer, in the short term at least, to treat the lesion with endovascular therapy or SRS, when appropriate, as opposed to surgery.
- **The age and general medical condition of the patient**: In general, older patients, particularly over the age of 75, or patients with multiple medical problems such as active heart, lung or kidney disease, or diabetes mellitus, are at higher risks of post-treatment complications.

- **The experience of the neurosurgeon**: The rate of complications "quoted" to a patient by his or her neurosurgeon should be his or her personal complication rates rather than those reflected in the literature, which may be higher or lower in comparison.
- **Previous treatment**: A brain lesion treated by previous open surgery or SRS or endovascular therapy may be associated with higher complication rates following subsequent treatment.

For the majority of brain conditions coming to open surgery, radiosurgery, or endovascular surgery, there is a 95% or better chance that treatment will be without significant complication. However, the final percentages are subject to discussion between the patient and the surgeon, and should take into consideration the factors mentioned above.

What types of treatment complications can occur?

Any complication a patient can think of can occur with any treatment. However, the chances of such complications occurring are usually low. Some general points are as follows:

- **Open surgical complications**: Certain complications apply to patients undergoing open surgery, as their treatment and postoperative care is usually more complex and prolonged compared with patients undergoing endovascular or radiosurgical treatment. General medical complications among patients undergoing open surgery include death under anesthesia from some very rare reaction to anesthetics. The chance of this is well under 1%. Other relatively rare complications include DVT, aspiration pneumonia, and PE. New seizures can also occur postoperatively. If any seizures do occur, they are usually temporary, lasting in the order of days to a few months. Major stroke or other brain tissue injury resulting in some permanent neurological disability such as impaired eyesight, double vision, speech and swallowing difficulty, facial and/or limb weakness or paralysis, incoordination and imbalance can also occur. A final and more specific discussion of the chances of any of these occurring is deferred to a patient's treating physician.

• **Complications of endoscopic neurosurgery**: Bleeding and infection are the main risks, but sometimes incomplete tumor removal occurs. In some instances, impairment of **memory** function can occur during navigation of the endoscope through the brain, with some form of injury to a structure known as the **fornix**. These risks should be discussed with the neurosurgeon.

• **WBRT and radiosurgical complications**: These include early **swelling and/or redness** around soft tissues of the scalp and/or face tissue through which the radiation beams have passed. It does *not* mean that the brain itself is swelling. Soft tissue swelling occurs fairly commonly after SRS, and usually in the first few days to a week following radiosurgery. It is **treated conservatively** with over-the-counter anti-inflammatory medications, walking about, and ice-packs. This sort of swelling typically begins to settle within a few days. If a head frame was used for SRS, the pin sites can swell and become red too. These findings do not necessarily imply infection, and should settle within a few days with conservative treatment as indicated above. If pus oozes from the pin sites, a patient should see his or her doctor. Some patients also complain of nausea and headaches soon after SRS, but these symptoms tend to settle on their own within days. **Hair loss** is very rare with SRS unless the lesion being treated is very close to the scalp. It may be more common with WBRT. If hair loss does occur with SRS, it is usually in a patch and will typically grow back. Hair loss with WBRT, and especially if additional chemotherapy is given, tends to be more diffuse and hair regrowth slower. Delayed swelling within the brain, referred to as **radiation necrosis**, is a potentially serious complication that can occur several months after radiation therapy. It occurs in some patients following radiation and can present with signs of raised ICP and any type of neurological deficit. It is frequently treated with steroids and sometimes by open surgery. WBRT and SRS can also **damage**

neighboring normal structures, including brain tissue and cranial nerves. For SRS, the radiation tends to taper off from the main target and into tissue in the vicinity of the radiation "field", albeit at a lower dose than for the target itself. **New neurological impairment**, which is unlikely to occur but can occur, should be reported to the doctor. For example, there may be delayed visual or hearing problems, or facial weakness, if the nerves for vision and hearing or facial muscle movement were near the primary radiation target. WBRT can cause **cognitive impairment** and, whenever possible, is avoided in younger persons. The other main complication of WBRT or radiosurgery is that it may **fail to control** the pathology for which it is being administered. For example, an irradiated tumor or AVM may continue to grow and/or cause problems despite SRS. It may be **radiation-resistant**. In very rare instances, a **second tumor** can form that may be the result of the radiation itself.

- **Endovascular complications**: These include infection and an expanding painful blood clot at the site of groin puncture, both of which are relatively uncommon. Other complications include a temporary neurological impairment or a permanent stroke at the time of catheter navigation and endovascular therapy. This can arise from an injury such as dissection or rupture of a vessel wall, or from unexpectedly extensive clot forming within the treated vessel territory, and sometimes breaking off to other parts of the brain circulation. In some cases, endovascular therapy may not fully treat the condition, and repeated endovascular surgery or open surgery may be required to complete the treatment.

- **Chemotherapy complications**: There are many different **side-effect profiles** for chemotherapy agents used alone or in some combination. Some are tolerated better by certain patients than others. As chemotherapy medications tend to **target rapidly dividing cells** that are typical of high grade tumors or cancers, and because some of the body's cells such as in the gut, skin and bone marrow are also rapidly dividing, chemotherapy agents also carry the potential to damage these normal cells. Relatively common side effects include nausea, vomiting, and gastrointestinal (GI) upset. There may be hair loss, particularly if the patient has both chemotherapy and radiation therapy. There is often some form of reduced white cell production referred to as leucopenia, and sometimes more generalized bone marrow impairment referred to as **myelosuppression** can occur. This can lead to reduced red blood cell production or **anemia**, and increased problems with infection and blood clotting. Chemotherapy agents can also damage organs in the body such as the kidney, liver, and heart. They may also damage the nerves of the limbs or peripheral nervous system, resulting in sensory and muscle or motor functional impairment from **peripheral neuropathy**. Rare severe toxic reactions to standard doses and combinations of chemotherapy agents have been reported. It is recommended that a chemotherapy patient's physician **regularly screen** the patient's blood for development of abnormalities in the complete blood count, and kidney and liver function tests. Finally, regarding brain chemotherapy implants such as **Gliadel® wafers**, brain swelling and local wound problems can occur with these, requiring their surgical removal.

• **Steroid complications**: Steroid therapy complications include high blood pressure or hypertension, sodium and fluid retention or damming in the body, GI upset or frank GI system disease, confusion, and elevated mood referred to as euphoria. **Cushing's syndrome** can also occur with long-term steroid use, usually in the order of months. This is associated with swelling of the face, increased facial and body hair, muscle wasting, weight gain, poor and bruised skin quality, hypertension, and so forth. Steroids can also cause **suppression of the immune system**, with increased likelihood of general infections, **poorer wound healing** and **wound infections**. In some instances, chronic steroid use can lead to muscle weakness and wasting known as steroid myopathy. The patient's white cell count can also rise with steroid use. Finally, abrupt stopping of steroids, that is, without true tapering or gradual weaning, in a patient who has been on steroids for at least several days can cause a syndrome of **steroid withdrawal** which includes nausea, vomiting, a feeling of generalized weakness and unwellness, and depression.

CHAPTER 19.

Recurrent or persistent disease after treatment, and the need for follow-up

A **recurrent lesion** is one that regrows after apparently successful treatment, that is, where the neurosurgeon thought that the lesion was obliterated by the procedure. On the other hand, a **persistent lesion** is one that continues to grow because the neurosurgeon was aware that it was not completely obliterated at the initial treatment attempt. Why wasn't it obliterated completely? The lesion may have been too large or too deep for the attempted treatment, or may have been too close to, or involving, a critical brain neurovascular structure. Finally, a **new lesion** is one that occurs in a different location to any other that was known and treated.

The chance of the same lesion recurring or regrowing after treatment really depends on two critical factors: (1) The **extent of surgical resection**; and (2) the **pathology of the lesion**. The former refers to how much of the lesion was physically removed or resected by the surgeon, while the latter refers to the exact type of lesion itself based on a pathologist's microscopic look at the cells making up the lesion.

Consider the following examples:

- **Brain aneurysm**: The chance of the same brain aneurysm growing is significantly higher if an endovascular surgeon or microneurosurgeon could not fully obliterate the aneurysm, that is, left a small corner or "dog ear" for whatever reason. In such situations, the chance of detecting ongoing growth in that aneurysm is around 1% per year. For endovascular treatment of larger aneurysms, that is, > 10 mm in diameter, the chance of the same aneurysm recurring or regrowing is somewhere between 25-50%, depending on the aneurysm's original size, and regardless of how well the endovascular treatment seemed to have gone. Of these aneurysms, about half can be effectively re-coiled, but the other half cannot. The latter are more frequently being referred to microneurosurgeons for treatment.

- **Benign brain tumor**: A benign brain tumor such as a **meningioma** is not expected to recur if it is entirely removed, that is, **gross totally resected**, along with the dura from which it arose. If the dura was left behind, or a small portion of tumor was left because it encased a critical blood vessel, the meningioma may certainly grow back. Frequently, this growth or regrowth is slow and can often be significantly retarded or stopped with SRS.

- **Malignant brain tumor**: A brain tumor such as a World Health Organization (WHO) grade 2, 3, or 4 **astrocytoma** is expected to recur even despite what appears to be a good resection based on the surgeon's intraoperative impression and the immediate postoperative MRI. The reason for this is that such tumors do not have distinct borders, and send small fingers of cells deeper throughout the neighboring brain. It is not possible at this time to remove every cell of an astrocytoma, although its growth or regrowth can be significantly slowed by a good resection followed by, where deemed appropriate, radiation therapy and chemotherapy. A high-grade astrocytoma such as **anaplastic astrocytoma** (WHO Grade 3 of 4) or **gliobastoma multiforme** (**GBM**; WHO Grade 4 of 4) is likely to grow or regrow more rapidly than a low-grade astrocytoma (WHO Grade 2 of 4). Untreated GBMs are thought to have overall size-doubling times of approximately one month, and despite multimodality treatment including surgery, radiation, and chemotherapy, have average survival times of approximately 12-15 months.

- **Chronic subdural hematoma** (SDH): A chronic SDH is a blood clot that has been sitting on the surface of a patient's brain for weeks or months. Such lesions develop membranes around them, and may have internal walls or loculations. They are notorious among neurosurgeons for being tricky to treat, and are commonly found to be persistent or recurrent despite surgical treatment.

It cannot be overstated that for all of the above reasons and scenarios, it is important that patients with brain conditions have appropriate clinical and radiological followup after treatment of the lesion. This means periodically scheduled Office visits with a physician, and surveillance imaging with, say, head CT or MRI/MRA. This issue should be discussed between the patient and physician prior to dismissal from hospital. Patients can certainly monitor their own symptom progression, and should report significant changes in their neurological state to their doctor.

Just because a patient has recurrent or persistent disease does not mean that there are no further treatment options. Certainly, some patients may be advised against further treatment, owing to, say, the extensive nature of their original disease, poor overall medical condition, or previous "maximal" therapy involving previous surgery, radiation and chemotherapy. However, others do have the options of, for example, repeat surgery and/or SRS where appropriate. For many patients, SRS can be used even if WBRT has been administered. **Salvage surgery** is a term that is sometimes used in the setting of a patient requiring repeated surgery for an advanced disease process. Some patients undergoing "salvage" treatments fare well, but others do not, despite heroic attempts by all concerned.

CHAPTER 20.
Recovery and rehabilitation

General comments on recovery

The road to recovery may be short or it may be a long one. For many, it is successfully traversed. For some, it is not. Others are given no fighting chance from the onset. The recovery period for "elective" treatment in patients with brain conditions is frequently shorter and less complex compared with that for patients undergoing "emergency" treatment.

Brain disorders can take their toll on a patient and his or her family members physically and psychologically. **Physically**, for a patient undergoing open surgery for a brain condition, there may be wound-related discomfort (**Chapter 16**) and fatigue. **Fatigue**, which may be described as feeling "drained" or "generally weak", can persist for a few months following hospitalization. It will likely resolve with time, but its resolution may be helped by regular napping and by eventually weaning off medications such as those for pain or seizures per the physician's recommendations. In addition, there may be **new physical impairment**(s) associated with the condition or its treatment, including problems with balance and coordination, weakness in one or more limbs, difficulty with speech and swallowing, and problems with vision. Many times, such deficits improve with time. They may resolve entirely, or partially. Physical healing may take a few or several months, even a few years, and may need PT. It is possible that a patient with a serious brain condition may permanently require assistance with his or her **activities**

of daily living (ADL), such as dressing, bathing, walking, eating, and so forth. **Psychologically,** for a patient, there may be problems associated with a depressed mood, emotional or behavioral instability, or slowed or abnormal brain processing referred to as **cognitive dysfunction.** Cognitive dysfunction may also include impairment of language and memory functions. All of the above may negatively impact on a patient's **sexual functioning** and sex drive. These psychological and cognitive problems may take months or a few years to improve and, again, their resolution may be complete or partial.

Family members of severe brain disorder survivors may come across times when they are forced to make very difficult decisions, and deal with circumstances that they may never have imagined before such an event. It is important that they remain strong, persistent, and united through this difficult time. The patient is likely facing a life-altering event, whose recovery frequently requires considerable patience and ongoing love and support, even if the event seems to have changed them physically and/or psychologically. Persons who survive severe brain injury or disease frequently **need more help** than they were previously used to or more than they may be willing to accept. Such help is critical and should benefit them significantly. It may be in the form of PT, speech therapy, a psychologist or psychiatrist, a home nurse, a temporary stay in a skilled nursing facility, rehabilitation center or a nursing home, more contact and support from family members and friends, more interaction with a priest or church, or an equivalent religious or spiritual person or group. Time and positivity are essential.

Recovery from a brain disorder is influenced by many factors, including the following:

- **Clinical presentation**: Perhaps first and foremost is the manner of a brain disorder patient's presentation. Some patients are neurologically devastated at the time of their presentation to hospital. Others are surprisingly well despite their underlying condition.
- **Experience and resources**: Important factors involved in a patient's recovery are the experience of the physicians and paramedical staff, and the resources of the hospital facility

at which the patient is treated. Again, these may not be in a patient's hands, but when considering elective treatment of a brain disorder, a patient should research the treating doctor or facility's backgrounds, even by word of mouth and the Internet. For complex brain conditions, having the procedure carried out in a large teaching center is probably in a patient's best interest. The quality of the hospital's rehabilitation service is also paramount, because it is that team of doctors and therapists who will optimize recovery once the neurosurgeon has done his or her part.

- **Psyche**: Finally, it can hardly be overstated that a patient's mindset is critical to healing. Part of one's personal role in recovery means staying focused on healing, being positive, understanding how precious the days and moments of one's life are, maintaining a healthy and balanced diet, walking and getting as much sunshine as one can, and continuing to meet with family and friends as regularly as possible. Returning to one's job, whenever possible, is a wonderful milestone to cross.

Will "alternative" therapies help a patient?

Alternative therapies are those that are not "mainstream", that is, neither surgical nor rehabilitation therapy. Although their definitions are somewhat subjective, today the divide between "mainstream" and "alternative" is narrowing. Alternative therapies include yoga, acupuncture, massage therapy, and hydrotherapy. However, hydrotherapy may be a part of a mainstream PT program. Do they help? Yes, they often help people, including brain disorder patients, in the healing process. Do they help all persons? No, not all, maybe not even most, but they definitely have helped some. Will they help a specific patient? No one can know this till he or she has tried one or more of these. Will they hurt? They are very unlikely to hurt a person in any significant way. One or more of these "alternative" therapies may be of benefit to patients if carried out in a professional and safe way by caring and appropriately trained individuals.

Rehabilitation

Many brain disorder patients will not require formal inpatient or outpatient rehabilitation. However, a significant proportion will. Rehabilitation services are available at most teaching hospitals, usually as part of a Department of PMR. Rehabilitation services represent an umbrella for a multitude of subdisciplines, and the "**rehab team**" is comprised of several members:

- **Physiatrists**: Physicians who have specialized in rehabilitation medicine and who **oversee** the rehabilitation process for patients admitted to their Service.
- **PTs**: Individuals who have special training in activities, both passive and active, that will improve a patient's **coordination, strength and balance**. PTs work on specific muscle group movements and exercises, and the patient as a whole. Some also train certain patients in the use of wheel chairs and walkers.
- **Occupational therapists** (OTs): Persons who work on activities that are directly relevant to a patient's **ADL**, such as bathing, toileting, dressing, navigating around the ward or through rooms in which a home-like environment is simulated, or in and out of a car. Some also train certain patients in the use of wheel chairs and walkers as they apply to navigating in a home environment, and engage patients in games and activities that focus on dexterity and concentration.
- **Speech therapists**: Persons who assess an individual's **speech and swallowing function**, both at the bedside and in an imaging suite. X-ray techniques are used for the formal assessment of swallowing function, and "dysphagia", "aspiration", and "laryngeal penetration" are terms commonly used as markers of swallowing impairment. Speech therapists focus on exercises that are geared towards improving speech and swallowing function which can be impaired particularly by lesions involving the brainstem and lower cranial nerves.
- **Social workers**: Individuals who assess the **social support networks** of a patient and provide information and coordination regarding **community support services** that may be of direct

benefit to certain patients. They assist in finding appropriate placement or **disposition** for certain patients who are ready to be dismissed from the hospital facility but are not yet ready to transition to a home environment. Placement may in a nursing home or a skilled nursing facility, or an acute rehabilitation facility closer to the patient's home.

- **Psychologists**: Persons trained in addressing the **psychological stresses and needs** of patients and their significant others. Specifically, they may assist in depression and behavioral counseling, and may provide important recovery strategies for patients with significant memory and cognitive impairment.
- **Rehabilitation nurses**: Nursing staff with a special interest in the well being of rehab patients.
- **Rehabilitation admission coordinators**: As the title suggests, rehab coordinators act as **liaisons** between hospital and insurance services and patients in the assessment of suitability for inpatient rehabilitation. Note that many rehab services have **specific criteria** that must be met for inpatient stay. Such criteria involve determining if a patient is neurologically impaired enough to require inpatient rehab, and if a patient requiring inpatient rehab is awake and interactive enough to meaningfully participate in, for example, a minimum of three hours per day of rehabilitation exercises and activities. Further, the patient's insurance should allow for inpatient rehabilitation. If the insurer does not permit this, for whatever reason, the request for transfer to the rehab unit can be denied. However, rehabilitation may still be permitted at a unit closer to the patient's home. Alternatively, special "charitable" funds may be available from the hospital, or the PMR and Neurosurgical Services may negotiate directly with an insurance company through the hospital to see if an appropriate arrangement can be made.

What can a patient expect regarding rehabilitation?

- **"Bedside rehab"**: Most patients with severe brain conditions will have bedside rehabilitation. This will typically begin with the assessment of a physiatrist, followed by the direct involvement of PTs, and possibly also OTs and a speech therapist. If a patient is comatose or semi-comatose, rehabilitation services can still be consulted mainly for two reasons: (1) Basic "**range of motion" (ROM) exercises**, which are commenced early to prevent or minimize loss of muscle bulk and development of joint contractures from disuse; and (2) having a PMR Service on board from an early stage in a critically ill or neurologically impaired patient is helpful for future inpatient rehabilitation planning. It should be noted that some Services may determine that a patient is physically and cognitively sound enough not to require any rehab, but will ask for formal assessment by PTs and OTs to assess the patient from the perspective of personal safety as they transition to home. This is referred to as a "**home safety assessment**". For example, can the patient get out of bed to a chair or walk a reasonable distance without falling? Can he or she get into a bath tub, dress independently, navigate around a room steadily, climb stairs, and eat without assistance? These therapists will provide invaluable advice to the patient regarding their home-going needs, including need for bath rails, ankle orthoses, walkers, wheelchairs, and so forth.

- "**Inpatient rehab**": Many brain disorder patients will undergo a period of inpatient rehabilitation. This will most often be at the facility at which they were admitted, but sometimes at a facility closer to their homes, or both. Once the Neurosurgery Service is satisfied that it has carried out everything it can for a patient, for patients who are still significantly neurologically impaired, the consulting PMR Service is requested to take over primary care. Such patients are transferred to the **PMR "floor" or "unit"** in the hospital. Here, all the team members of the PMR Service can interact with the patient in a closer and more personal manner. In this environment, the patient has direct access to the various rehab programs and resources. The inpatient stay in rehab varies from patient to patient according to their physical, cognitive and psychosocial needs. It is usually a minimum of one week, and may be for several weeks. The exercises and activities involved in the unit include those mentioned above. Dismissal from a rehab facility usually entails a determination that the patient is now strong, mentally sound, and safe enough to transition to the home environment. If not, the patient may be dismissed to another rehab or other type of facility closer to his or her home according to the patient's needs.

- **"Outpatient rehab"**: This is generally for patients who have been through, or are in too good a neurologic condition for, inpatient rehab. Such patients are set up with community PTs, typically closer to their home. Outpatient PT sessions may be as frequent as once daily or as infrequent as once weekly following dismissal. **Instructions** are usually provided in the dismissal summary or in a specific referral letter from the hospital physiatrist. The duration of outpatient rehab varies from patient to patient. It may be for a few weeks or a few months. The primary doctor should **reassess** the patient somewhere within 3 months of surgery and at that time make any further recommendations for ongoing PT needs, if any. Many PTs in the community wish to have a written prescription or referral letter or detailed dismissal summary from the primary doctor or hospital Service specifying the duration and type of outpatient PT required.

CHAPTER 21.

Four case histories (brain tumors, brain hemorrhage, brain trauma)

The following four brief patient stories represent scenarios that can occur with brain tumors, hemorrhage, and trauma. Pseudonyms have been used.

M.K., Low grade brain tumor

Following 3 weeks of unexplained morning headaches, M.K., a 42-year old man, went to his local doctor. He had no vomiting or nausea, no seizures, simply headaches. His local doctor found M.K. to have a normal neurological exam, but ordered a plain CT head scan. This showed a 4 cm diameter lesion or mass located in the right hemisphere, in the frontal lobe, and there appeared to be mild swelling or "shift" associated with it. To better define the lesion, M.K.'s doctor ordered a brain MRI, with and without contrast. This study showed the lesion in better detail. The lesion only very faintly took up the contrast agent, was round overall with some irregular margins, and appeared to be a solid mass. The radiologist suspected this was a primary brain tumor, most likely a glioma such as an astrocytoma. M.K. was given a prescription for oral steroid to assist in reducing the brain swelling, and expeditiously referred to a neurosurgeon.

The neurosurgeon agreed that this was most likely an astrocytoma, probably a "low grade" one given that it didn't really enhance or light up with the contrast dye. He described the 4 grades of astrocytoma according to the WHO classification, with M.K.'s lesion most likely a WHO grade 2 astrocytoma. The surgeon also went over the treatment options. It was explained that this kind of lesion with its appearance and symptom was not one to observe. It was located in a relatively safe part of the brain, and that surgical removal was the preferable first-line treatment compared with radiation therapy or chemotherapy. The procedure, called a right-side frontotemporal craniotomy and resection, was explained in detail to M.K. and his wife, as were the risks, benefits, alternatives, and so forth. The neurosurgeon opted to use a stereotactic image-guidance system for the surgery, which would allow him to plan a relatively small incision and craniotomy, and resect the tumor as safely and completely as possible. The surgeon's preference would be to ask the anesthesiologist to administer an anti-seizure medication during surgery, and a dose of steroid. It was anticipated that the steroid would be weaned soon after surgery, but the anti-seizure medicine would be maintained for several weeks after surgery, and then weaned under the supervision of M.K.'s local doctor.

Surgery was carried out and was uneventful. M.K. awoke with no neurological impairment, and spent one night in the neuro-ICU where he was closely observed. The following morning, he underwent a postoperative brain MRI, which showed a **gross total resection** (GTR), implying complete resection by imaging. The neurosurgeon explained to M.K. that even though the scan looked fine, owing to the way astrocytomas grew, at a microscopic level, there were tumor cells still present in the surrounding brain region, and therefore he should be mindful of the scenario of further treatment, including the possibility of repeated surgery, some time down the road, maybe several years away.

M.K. was transferred to the neurosurgical general care ward. He was able to walk independently the next morning, and although he had some incisional pain, this was for the most part well controlled with narcotic pain medications. As he was neurologically intact, no rehabilitation was necessary. The pathology specimens sent from the OR returned as low grade astrocytoma, and the brain tumor physicians or neuro-oncologists were consulted by the neurosurgical team to advise regarding postoperative radiation and chemotherapy. Their advice was to let M.K. recover from the surgery, and to obtain another surveillance MRI in 3 months. They felt that because of the pathology and the tumor's GTR, M.K. could be observed with serial scans. At the first sign of the tumor's return radiologically, he would receive radiation therapy and chemotherapy. He was dismissed from hospital 3 days after surgery.

Twelve days after surgery, M.K.'s scalp staples were removed and he was found to be doing very well. At the 3 month postoperative visit, M.K. continued to be doing very well. He was without neurological symptoms or impairment, and had no spells or seizures. There was no evidence of tumor regrowth on the 3 month MRI study. M.K.'s seizure medications were weaned over the subsequent 3 weeks. Another scan was organized for 6 months down the road with followup by the neurooncologist.

L.S., High grade brain tumor

L.S., a 57-year old man, was brought to the ER by his family because he had progressively developed speech difficulties and unsteadiness with falls. The neurologist who examined L.S. found him to be mildly confused, verified that he did indeed have a speech disorder or aphasia, and that he was mildly weak on the right side, with obvious gait imbalance. A CT scan of the head showed a large mass situated in the temporal lobe, extending up through the frontal lobe on the left side. An MRI was ordered, with and without contrast, to better define the mass. This showed that the mass, which measured 6 cm in its largest diameter, had an irregular and shaggy border that lit up with contrast, in the form of a ring. The lesion was causing significant "mass effect" and threatened to cause herniation. A neurosurgeon was consulted. The physicians communicated to the patient and his family that this was most likely a primary tumor of high grade because of its appearance. A secondary or metastatic tumor was also possible, though less likely, and an infection or brain abscess was much less likely per the MRI and the patient's presentation. The neurosurgeon explained that this was a serious situation, given the impending herniation, and that the option representing the best interests of the patient was to undergo a craniotomy with debulking of the mass. He explained that surgery would establish the diagnosis for appropriate treatment planning, as well as relieve the mass effect, which would otherwise soon become a life-threatening issue if unchecked. The risks of the procedure were explained, including further problems to speech and movement, in addition to the possibility of vision problems as part of the visual pathways bordered the mass. However, the benefits of surgery clearly and significantly outweighed the risks.

L.S. was taken to the operating room, and underwent the craniotomy and resection as planned, without any perceived problems intraoperatively according to the neurosurgeon. Owing to the large size of the mass, the neurosurgeon elected to keep L.S. intubated overnight in the ICU. The surgeon explained to the family that the mass appeared to be a primary brain tumor or glioma, most likely a high-grade astrocytoma as suggested by the pathologist's frozen section specimen results communicated to the team during the surgery. He added that such tumors could not be fully removed, but he was able to get the majority of the mass out. The neurooncologists were consulted when the final diagnosis from the specimen returned as WHO grade 4 of 4 fibrillary astrocytoma or GBM, unfortunately the highest grade of brain tumor.

L.S. was extubated 24 hours after surgery. His postoperative MRI scan showed a good but not total resection, although there was significant swelling around the operative bed. He was weaker on the right side than he was before surgery, and the surgical team put him on high-dose steroids to help reduce the swelling that they thought was responsible for this decline. The PMR Service was consulted, and PT and OT therapy at the bedside begun. After a few days, L.S. was considered stable enough to transfer to the neurosurgical general ward, and after a few more days was transferred to the rehab unit of the hospital, where he continued to improve and was dismissed 2 weeks after the operation.

The neurooncologists who visited with the patient and his family advised that for GBM, the best possible chance of survival was with both postoperative radiation therapy and chemotherapy. They recommended a 6-week course of brain radiation commencing 3 weeks after surgery, and Temozolamide chemotherapy. L.S. underwent both, and was seen regularly by members of the radiation and medical oncology services throughout this time.

Unfortunately, and as seen in most patients with GBM, despite aggressive surgery and postoperative treatments, L.S.'s GBM began to regrow within 6 months of the initial diagnosis. He had once again become more confused and weak. The only viable option at this time was salvage surgery to debulk some of the mass, although the medical oncologists suggested that a chemotherapy agent in the form of a Gliadel® wafer could be left in the tumor bed at the time of repeat surgery, to provide local anti-tumor therapy. However, the family declined further treatment, as they felt that L.S. had been through enough, and that his overall prognosis was poor. The neurosurgeon suggested that a shunt could be placed to allow the CSF pathways to remain as viable as possible, given the recurrent swelling in the brain, but the family again declined for understandable reasons. L.S. passed away seven months after the initial diagnosis in a hospice facility under the close watch of his supportive family. His family reported that he experienced no obvious pain, he just became sleepier.

F.D., Brain hemorrhage

F.D., a 61-year old independent and active woman with known high blood pressure, was unfortunately noncompliant with her medications in that she did not take them regularly. She was brought by ambulance to the ER having collapsed at her home in the presence of her family. She was poorly responsive at the time of her evaluation in the ER, and was noted to have weakness on her left side. A CT scan of the head revealed a 4 cm bleed in the right side of the brain, with some shift of the midline structures from the hematoma's mass effect. The neurosurgery team felt that removing the hematoma would be appropriate, given its location and the shift. The neurosurgeon explained that the procedure would be a life-saving procedure, and that he anticipated F.D. would have some, possibly significant, residual weakness on the left side owing to the location of the hemorrhage. He added that, despite postoperative rehab, she might still remain considerably dependent on others in her

ADL. The family wanted the neurosurgery team to be as aggressive as possible, and F.D. was accordingly taken to the OR after informed consent was received.

The surgeon reported that the operation went uneventfully and that the intraoperative pathology was consistent with a hematoma from a hypertensive hemorrhage. F.D. was extubated the following day, and was appropriately following commands despite stable weakness of her left side. Her postoperative head CT scan looked fine, the hematoma had been entirely evacuated. The PMR service was consulted, and bedside rehab was commenced. F.D. had recovered enough to transfer to the neurosurgery general care ward a few days later and then, per her family's request, was moved to a rehab facility closer to their home. Her 2-week postoperative CT scan and wound check were fine, and it was recommended by the neurosurgeon that she have long-term rehabilitation, for weeks as an inpatient, and then for months as an outpatient. This was carried out.

Six months postoperatively, F.D. had made good gains in her strength. Although her left side was by no means normal, she could walk with the aid of a framed walker and mild assistance of a companion, and was able to do some of her ADL with only a mild amount of assistance and supervision. The neurosurgeon reassured F.D. and her family that she would continue to make gains over the next several months, and recommended further outpatient rehab therapy. F.D.'s hypertension was now being tightly controlled by her local internist, and she had become fully compliant with her therapy.

K.L., Brain trauma

At the age of 16, K.L. was involved in a motor vehicle accident. She was not wearing a seatbelt and was ejected from the overturned vehicle. Fortunately, ground and air paramedics got to her soon after the accident. She was unconscious at the scene but breathing, had obvious head and limb injuries, and was intubated for her helicopter flight back to the hospital. The ER was alerted about her condition *en route*, and the full Trauma Team was mobilized for her arrival. A general surgeon, ER specialist, orthopedic surgeon, and neurosurgeon rapidly assessed her top to toe upon her arrival, and the usual blood tests and imaging studies were rapidly carried out. Despite having sustained several rib fractures, a broken arm and leg, moderate lung injuries and a small laceration of her liver, her spine CT showed no fracture or dislocation. Her head CT showed a small blood clot on the surface of her brain, a few areas of brain tissue bruising, a nondisplaced skull fracture, some brain swelling, but no major life-threatening brain injury. She was taken to the trauma ICU, however, the surgeons elected to place an EVD in the right side of K.L.'s brain to allow her ICP to be monitored and treated as needed. This was because her neurological exam was unreliable owing to the sedatives and muscle relaxants she had on board, and also because the orthopedic surgeons would need to take K.L. to the OR for her fractures. Having an EVD in place would provide some degree of monitoring for K.L.'s brain throughout the orthopedic procedure. Emergency consent for the EVD placement was obtained by two of the neurosurgeons in the absence of any relatives or other contacts.

Repeat head CT scanning later that evening showed that some of the bruises and small hematomas had "blossomed" into larger ones, but still none required open neurosurgery at that stage. K.L.'s ICP had remained normal, and when brought out of her medically induced coma, she was able to move her unfractured limbs. K.L. remained in a critical condition, intubated for 6 days. She had a feeding tube placed for her nutrition, and fortunately was safely extubated a day or two before it would have become necessary to place a tracheostomy. The PMR service assisted with bedside ROM activities, and the neurosurgery service removed K.L.'s EVD 24 hours after her extubation. She was able to follow commands intermittently, moved her unfractured limbs spontaneously, and at times opened her eyes and spoke to her family. An MRI of the brain had been carried out prior to her extubation, and this showed DAI-type shear injury to several areas of the brain, implying a need for months to heal. A short time later, K.L.'s feeding tube was removed after a formal video-assisted swallowing study showed that she could swallow without any significant aspiration.

The TBI rehab doctors were consulted, and once K.L. had recovered significantly from her acute injuries, she was transferred to the inpatient rehab unit for further care and therapy. She remained on this unit for more than six weeks, and was eventually dismissed to home, with a provision made for ongoing outpatient rehab therapy, including for PT, OT, speech, and neuropsychology. With the support of her family, her own personal dedication, and the help of several medical and paramedical specialists, it still took almost 12 months for K.L. to return to a state resembling her pre-accident baseline.

CHAPTER 22.
Neurosurgery: What's on the horizon?

There are many exciting prospects on the neurosurgical horizon, each aimed at advancing patient care:

- **Advanced biomedical imaging** (BMI): Brain imaging techniques are becoming more sophisticated and their relatively recent evolution has made an enormous and positive impact upon patient diagnosis, care and outcome. **Functional imaging techniques** which not only examine brain structure, but also its functions such as regional blood flow and metabolism, and its biochemical signatures, are likely going to be of major significance with time. Still evolving techniques include MRS, functional MRI (fMRI), PET, and intraoperative fluorescence microscopy. The OR environment in many centers is also becoming more advanced, with **real-time intraoperative MRI** becoming more available, and a **film-free hospital environment** becoming a reality. **Intraoperative image guidance** using infrared and laser technology represents a major advance in surgical accuracy and safety, as the surgeon is guided by his or her instruments or microscope lasers with precision through the brain and to the lesion. In the OR, **large split-screens** simultaneously projecting the real-time view under the operating microscope, the preoperative brain imaging, and the intraoperative image-guidance view are starting to be installed in centers. **Wireless technology** is also making its mark on the ability of physicians to confidentially access their patients' studies, including imaging, using handheld and laptop devices. A newer technique known as **diffusion tensor imaging** (DTI) may also become more widely incorporated into the OR. DTI allows for imaging of important pathways such as the corticospinal tract (CST) responsible for movement of the opposite of the body. The information obtained from DTI can be used in the OR, including in 3D, so that a lesion close to, say, the CST can be removed with more precision, as the imaging data allows the surgeon to see where he or she is operating relative to the location of the CST.

- **Virtual reality technology** (VRT): The age of real-time immersion of surgeons into a realistic electronic environment is dawning through advances in VRT. The ability to carry out surgery remotely, that is, where the surgeon is not in the same immediate environment as the patient, has already been successfully demonstrated in the fields of general and cardiac surgery. It remains to be seen whether this type of surgery, referred to as **telesurgery**, will become a practice among neurosurgeons treating patients in geographically remote areas or in a makeshift hospital on a battlefield, or in outer space (**Figure 28**). Advances in VRT are also enabling surgeons to practice complex surgical approaches prior to the actual operation itself, through realistic, **textured, 3D imaging software** coupled to desktop computers and hand-held instruments. Finally, the incorporation of a patient's **ghosted brain imaging** into the eyepieces of the surgeon's image-guided operating microscope, similar to technology already available to air force pilots, is anticipated to make a positive contribution to operative safety and success.

- **Robotics**: Computer-controlled robotic arms are already being used for precision delivery of radiation (as in the **Cyberknife®** SRS system) and in the setting of **functional neurosurgery** where stimulating probes are inserted into deep brain structures. The further development of **telesurgery** will necessarily require hand-in-hand advances in telerobotics, because it will be the remote robotic arms and cameras carrying out the surgery according to the surgeon's feedback and hand movements (**Figure 28**).

- **Genetic technologies**: Using blood and tissue tests to diagnose medical conditions based on their unique genetic signatures is already a reality. Developing and using **genetic screening techniques** or assays based on simple blood samples to predict the development or outcome of brain conditions is an emerging reality. This represents the anticipated benefits of the **Human Genome Project**, and the current **genomics and proteomics revolutions**. Further, ongoing advances in the field of **gene therapy** will likely, in time, allow a variety of CNS conditions to be effectively treated by appropriate delivery of gene-based medicines aimed at specifically correcting defects at a genetic or molecular level, or at targeting tumor and other abnormal cells while preserving normal brain cells. The fields of genomics, proteomics and gene therapy are overviewed elsewhere (**www.brain-aneurysm.com**).

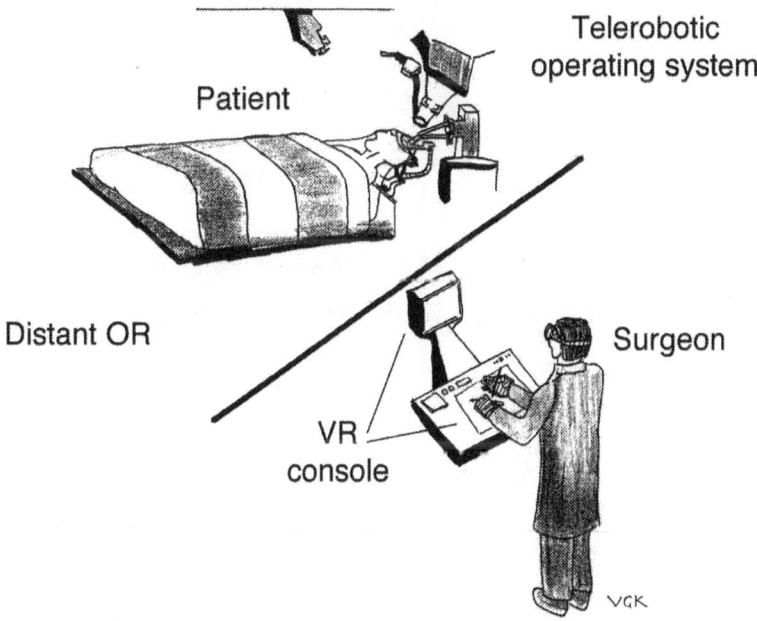

Figure 28. Telesurgery: The OR telesuite.

CHAPTER 23.

The brain disorder and surgery checklist

SYMPTOMS & SIGNS:	Sudden onset of most severe headache
	Sudden neurological impairment: vision, speech, limbs
	Unexplained headaches (especially morning)
	Unexplained nausea, vomiting, drowsiness
	Unexplained headaches with fever and neck stiffness
	Progressive deafness or ringing in one ear, vertigo, gait imbalance
	Progressive neurological changes (any of the above)
	Miscellaneous: Seizure, personality and memory changes
INVESTIGATIONS:	CT head scan – low resolution study; good start to screen for lesions
	MRI head scan – high resolution study; good for most brain lesions

	MRA/V head and/or neck – to look at brain and neck arteries and veins
	CTA/V head and/or neck – to look at brain and neck arteries and veins
	Cerebral angiogram – high detail study of brain artery and vein roadmap
	PET scan – for brain blood flow and metabolism
	SPECT – for brain blood flow and brain blood volume
	TCD – for blood flow in brain arteries threatened by spasm
	Carotid ultrasound – for blood flow across the neck's carotid arteries
	Lumbar puncture – to obtain CSF for lab studies, spinal fluid pressure
	Blood tests – for markers of inflammation, infection; sodium; genetics
	Brain biopsy – brain tissue samples for pathology, microbiology (bugs)
TREATMENT OPTIONS:	Observation – periodic scans and Office visits but no active treatment
	Medical management – steroids, anti-seizure and pain meds, blood thinners
	Open surgery – major procedure: Craniotomy
	Open surgery – minor procedure: EVD, shunt, reservoir, needle biopsy
	Endovascular surgery – coils, stents, glues or resins

	Radiation therapy – whole-brain versus stereotactic
	Chemotherapy
INFORMED CONSENT:	Benefits of procedure
	Risks of procedure
	Overview of procedure
	Alternatives to the procedure
	Team approach
	Discussion of advance directives
HEALING:	Takes time, maybe several months
	May affect thinking clarity, personality, strength, agility, sexual function
	May involve formal rehabilitation therapy, speech therapist, psychologist
	Personal motivation, patience and psyche very important
	Social supports: family, friends, community resources; spiritual person or group
	Awareness that patients, family members are under new, extraordinary stresses
	Accept help
FOLLOW-UP:	Wound-check date
	Periodic Office visits
	Periodic scans
	Physician/Office contact numbers – write names, numbers down before leaving

CHAPTER 24.
Online resources

There is a lot of information on the Web. The following links are listed to provide the reader with helpful and comprehensive information about specific disorders of the brain, spinal cord and spine, and their treatments. It should be remembered that this information is not intended to take the place of personal consultation with a physician. For many more links, including updated links that may have changed in the interim, please visit **www.brain-surgery.us**, the official Website for this book.

URL:	DESCRIPTION:
http://neurosurgery.mgh.harvard.edu	This Site by the Harvard Medical School and the Massachusetts General Hospital has numerous links to explore regarding the spectrum of CNS disorders and their treatments.
http://www.ninds.nih.gov	An official and very comprehensive Site of the National Institutes of Health (NIH) and National Institute of Neurological Disorders and Stroke (NINDS). The Site has an A-Z disorder index.
http://hope.abta.org	Home of the American Brain Tumor Association. Information and links.

http://www.brain-aneurysm.com	A comprehensive, illustrated Site about brain blood vessel disorders by Dr. Khurana. The Site includes information on brain aneurysms, cerebral vasospasm, AVMs, carotid artery disease, venous angioma, cavernoma, gene therapy and genomics. Many educational radiological and operative images are also shown.
http://www.strokeassociation.org	Home of the American Stroke Association.
http://www.mayoclinic.com/health/nervous-system/BN99999	A Site about CNS disorders and specialist services by the Mayo Clinic. Search by disease or symptom.
http://www.thebni.com	The Barrow Neurological Institute's Homepage, with links to a variety of CNS diseases and specialist services.
http://www.brainaustralia.org.au	An informative Site by the Australian Brain Foundation.
http://www.ucsfhealth.org	Click the Health Library and Medical Services links of this Site belonging to the University of California at San Francisco.
http://www.spineuniverse.com	A Site with many links regarding disorders of the spine and their treatment.
http://www.brain-surgery.us	This "brain surgery help" Site has many helpful links for persons with brain disorders.
http://www.elekta.com/healthcareus.nsf	Homepage of the Gammaknife® makers.
http://www.accuray.com	Homepage of the Cyberknife® makers.
http://brain.mgh.harvard.edu/ChemoGuide.htm	A Harvard chemotherapy Site with links.
http://info.med.yale.edu/btumor/patients/chemoguide.html	A chemotherapy guide from Yale.

CHAPTER 25.
Some frequently asked questions (FAQs)

Here are some responses to questions frequently put to neurosurgeons by their patients.

Is my astrocytoma a cancer?

This is sometimes a very difficult question to answer. Unfortunately, there are few benign brain tumors, that is, tumors that can be confidently and effectively cured by brain surgery and/or additional therapies. Most brain tumors are malignant, akin to cancers, in that they tend to grow or regrow even despite initially adequate-appearing therapy. However, the rate of growth and the time to regrowth can vary incredibly. Malignant tumors cause disability and death by their continued growth, invasion and effects on adjacent brain structures. With the exception of pilocytic astrocytomas (WHO grade 1), adult astrocytomas are usually malignant, that is, they represent a form of brain cancer. Having stated this, however, it should be noted that some neurosurgeons prefer to think of low grade astrocytomas (WHO grade 2) as not being a cancer. This may be misleading. Although the survival from a WHO grade 2 astrocytoma is often measured in several or many years, these lesions are typically not curable, and will often transform into a higher grade astrocytoma with the passage of time. None-the-less, a patient should always remember that the statistics can be, and have been, beaten by many a person with a brain tumor. One should think of the diagnosis more as a battle, with victory favoring the brave, equipped and determined.

Will the aneurysm grow back after it's treated?

If the neurosurgeon or endovascular surgeon feels that the aneurysm has been obliterated based on the intraoperative or postoperative angiogram, the chance of it recurring or regrowing is very low, but still not zero. If there was a known residual or remnant, that is, a part of the aneurysm that remained unobliterated for whatever reason, then the chance of it recurring is increased. It is also possible that an entirely separate aneurysm can form in the same patient. For these reasons, appropriate radiological follow-up is mandatory for patients with brain aneurysms, even after apparently successful treatment. This should be discussed in detail with the surgeon.

What would you do if I were a close relative of yours?

The neurosurgeon will typically provide the best possible advice to his or her patient, and in the patient's best interests. That is, the advice he or she gives to the patient should be the same as he or she would have given to a loved one with the same condition.

Where will the incision be?

The incision is usually entirely hidden behind the hairline. For frontotemporal and pterional craniotomies, the incision starts just in front of the ear, ascends upwards behind the side hairline, and curves gently forwards towards the midline, at the top of the front part of the head, again, behind the top hairline. For a suboccipital craniotomy, the incision is within the hair-bearing part of the scalp in or near the midline at the back of the head, just above the neck. For a retrosigmoid craniotomy, the incision curves behind the ear, again, in the hair-bearing scalp. Other incisions may be anywhere and of various shapes and sizes in the hair-bearing scalp, depending on the site and size of the lesion being operated upon, and the surgeon's preferred approach. The surgeon will be able to trace out the incision for the patient at his or her request.

How much hair will you shave?

Many neurosurgeons are turning to the "minimal head shave" as a preferred approach. Where once it was typical to shave the whole side of a patient's head for surgery, it is now becoming more common that only a thin strip of hair is shaved. The strip is usually 1-1.5 cm, or approximately 0.5 inch, wide. The hair regrows.

How long will the surgery take?

The surgery will take as long as needed for the surgeon to safely and effectively accomplish the planned task. Most craniotomies take between 3 to 5 hours of "operating time", the time taken to carry out the physical part of the surgery itself. Shunt placement frequently takes less than one hour of operating time. Stereotactic biopsies usually take less than one-half hour of operating time. Endovascular surgery typically takes 1 to 3 hours of operating time, while SRS may take less than one hour of actual radiation time. However, the actual operating time is not the total time. The total time is that from when a patient is brought to the OR or procedure suite until the patient returns to the ICU. This time is made up of many "time intervals". These include the time taken to put the patient to sleep in the OR, the time taken to carefully pad, position, pinion, and prepare the patient prior to incision, the operating time itself, the time taken to wake the patient up, and the time to "recover" the patient in Recovery, and then transfer the patient to the ICU or ward. Therefore, despite an operating time frequently measured in a few hours, the time of surgery is frequently half a day. There should be some means of communication between the surgical team and the patient's family to periodically inform concerned relatives of the patient's progress throughout this stressful time.

Will I be in pain after open surgery?

Open brain surgery involves a scalp incision, and by definition this will cause pain. However, the pain is typically very well controlled by the use of IV followed by oral narcotic pain medications. There are plenty of medications available to assist, and a Pain Service can also help out when needed. Postoperative pain is not only related to the operation, it is also related to the patient's own "pain threshold". Regardless, the vast majority of brain surgery patients are successfully treated in terms of pain control. Pain improves daily, and within 7-10 days of surgery, most patients have begun to wean off their oral pain medications.

How long will I be in hospital?

Most elective or planned open brain surgery patients stay in the ICU for one or two nights, and then transition to a general neurosurgical ward for another 2-3 nights. If there is a complication, or if the patient is in poor neurological condition to begin with, as is often the case with neurosurgical emergencies, these calculations are of course subject to change. Most endovascular surgery patients are in hospital for only one or two nights. SRS patients typically leave the same day as the treatment itself. If inpatient rehab is needed because of the patient's serious brain condition, the stay could be a few to several weeks.

When will the staples or sutures come out?

This varies from surgeon to surgeon, but most surgeons desire them to be removed by 10-12 days after surgery. If the sutures were buried under the skin surface and small plastic Steristrips were applied to the skin surface, surgeons desire these strips to be removed no later than 7 days after surgery. A wound check appointment date with the neurosurgeon or with the patient's local doctor or nurse should be organized prior to the patient's dismissal from hospital.

Will the metal plates set off airport security detectors or stop me from getting an MRI?

Titanium miniplates and screws are typically used by neurosurgeons to restore the skull bone flap after a craniotomy, or to plate fractured bone in the setting of traumatic skull injuries. These do not set off airport metal detectors, nor do they interfere with the patient getting an MRI in the future. This also holds true for the wide array of modern day titanium brain aneurysm clips, and platinum microcoils and stents. A patient should always inform the radiologist before an MRI regarding any metal implants.

When can I return to my usual activities after surgery?

Patients are encouraged to return to walking and climbing stairs as soon as possible after surgery. Regarding activities such as sex and sports, patients are encouraged to "listen to themselves", that is, when their bodies tell them that it is okay to do so, they should do so. Driving is frequently a special concern, and this issue may be a complicated one if the patient has had seizures. In the setting of seizures, return to driving should be discussed with the neurosurgeon and neurologist. There are state-dependent guidelines regarding this, and the U.S. Department of Motor Vehicles Website can also be consulted for further information, as can the Epilepsy Foundation Website (http://www.epilepsyfoundation.org/answerplace/Legal/transit/drivelaw). In the absence of seizures, as long as there is no physical or mental impairment, it should be safe to return to driving when the patient and his family feel that it is safe enough to do so. Other specific activity restrictions may apply, for example, in the case of a patient who has sustained a significant TBI. These types of restrictions should be discussed with the physician.

When can I come off the anti-seizure medicines?

If a patient has experienced seizures as part of his or her medical condition and/or treatment, anti-seizure medications will typically be prescribed. The type(s) of medication and the length of treatment vary on a case-by-case basis. Also, some of these medications will need to have their blood levels periodically monitored by the patient's prescribing or local doctor to ensure that the drug remains at an effective level, that is, not too high nor too low. For patients on such medicines for a longer term, such as months, an electroencephalogram (EEG) will typically be ordered prior to tapering off or weaning the medication(s), as long as the patient has remained seizure-free during this treatment time. If the EEG shows no seizure-like or epileptiform activity, the medication is generally weaned over a period of weeks. The patient's prescribing physician should outline a plan for the patient regarding how long the medication is anticipated to be taken, who will check the patient's drug levels and when, and who will supervise the eventual weaning of such medications. If there are any doubts, the patient should clarify these with his or her prescribing physician. It is generally recommended that, owing to the possibility of a seizure occurring while weaning a seizure medication, the patient not drive or climb ladders, nor operate heavy machinery or engage in activities that could threaten his or her life or the lives of others, during the weaning period.